The Local BABY Directory™

Surrey & S. Middlesex

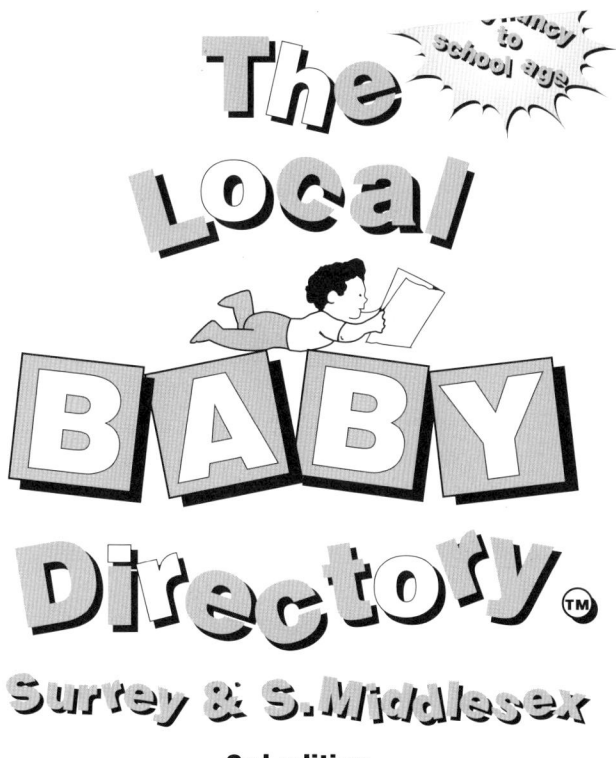

pregnancy to school age

3rd edition

An A-Z of EVERYTHING
for
pregnant women, babies and children

edited by
Angela Thompson

Disclaimer
While every effort has been made to verify the information provided, The Local Baby Directory (Surrey & S. Middlesex) can accept no responsibility for any inaccuracies or omissions. Inclusion in the Directory does not imply an endorsement of the service or product.

First published 2000
Second edition updated 2001
Third edition updated 2002

The Local Baby Directory
15 Lincoln Avenue, Twickenham, Middlesex TW2 6NH. 020 8898 2411

ISBN 1-903288-09-6

© Karen Liebreich

All rights reserved. No part of this publication may be reproduced or transmitted in any form, or by any means, electronic, mechanical, photocopying, recording or otherwise, or stored in any retrieval system, without prior written permission of the publisher.
The Data Protection Act requires that we inform you that if your company or service is listed in the Directory, it is on our computer.
Data Protection Register No: PX 4379316

lb⁄

Designed by LB Graphics, 01795 428150
Printed and bound in Great Britain by AOK Printers & Stationers, 01689 891460

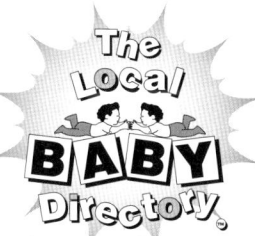

*The Local Baby Directory: Surrey & South Middlesex
covers:*
all of Surrey and the postal county of South Middlesex including the towns and surrounding areas of Ashford, Brentford, Feltham, Hampton, Hounslow, Isleworth, Teddington, Twickenham and Staines.

*Other Local Baby Directories now available:
Bristol, Bath & Somerset
Herts & Middlesex
Oxfordshire, Berks & Bucks
South Wales
Sussex & Hampshire
and*
The London Baby Directory

*Franchise possibilities
If there is no Baby Directory in your area and you think there should be,
contact us to discuss franchise opportunities.*

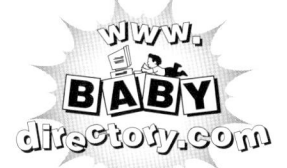

Visit our website for
■ The Baby Directory Encyclopaedia of Pregnancy & Birth ■
■ Medical Advice ■ Breastfeeding ■
■ Educational Advice ■
■ Nanny Agency ■
■ Book Shop ■ Prizes ■ Updates ■

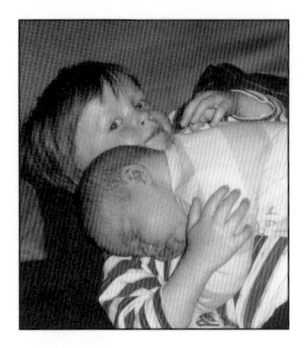

Biography

Angela has had another son, Johnny, a brother for Ross since the last edition of the Local Baby Directory was published. Although Johnny is still a bit small he will soon be joining Ross and enjoying many of the activities/goods/services listed in the Baby Directory. Some of Ross's favourites include swimming lessons, gym club and music classes. They've all had fun on lots of outings including trips to farms, indoor adventure playgrounds and parks. Ross is looking forward to introducing Johnny to all of his favourite toy shops and restaurants and he'll be bound to recommend his friendly homeopath should Johnny ever feel under the weather!

Acknowledgements

Karen without whom there would be no directory. **Sioux** for her fabulous design skills and great eye for colour. **Brigid, Janie** and **Gail** my fellow editors in crime. **Violet** for her creative drawings, **Hazel** for her help with our advertisers. **Pete** and his team for printing the books. **Ross** and **Johnny** for their help in research. **Paul** for looking after Ross and Johnny while I worked on the Baby Directory!

Welcome to the third edition of The Local Baby Directory: Surrey & South Middlesex – an A-Z reference source of pregnancy, baby and child related activities, services and retail outlets throughout the Surrey & South Middlesex area. This is a sister to the very successful London Baby Directory and Local Baby Directories in Bristol, Bath & Somerset, Herts & Middlesex, Beds, Bucks & Oxon, Sussex & Hampshire & South Wales.

Our aim is to provide you with one convenient source of local information for all your needs whilst pregnant or as a parent or carer with a baby, toddler or young child.

We have made no quality judgements about the entrants. The advertisers paid to be included. Any omissions from the directory are either oversights on our behalf or where we have been unable to verify the information. The accuracy of the listings has been checked to the best of our ability and we apologise for any mistakes that may have occurred. If you find any mistakes or omissions, or have any comments, please let us know by completing the feedback form.

Our website at **www.babydirectory.com** includes an Encyclopaedia of Pregnancy & Birth as well as updated listings for the whole of the UK, free medical advice, an excellent book shop, breastfeeding advice & a nanny agency.

We hope you find this Local Baby Directory useful.

Angela Thompson
Editor

NOTES

The Local Baby Directory - *Surrey & S. Middlesex*   www.babydirectory.com

notes to advertisers

Contact us for further details:
020 8898 2411
E-mail: a_j_thompson@hotmail.com
or see feedback page

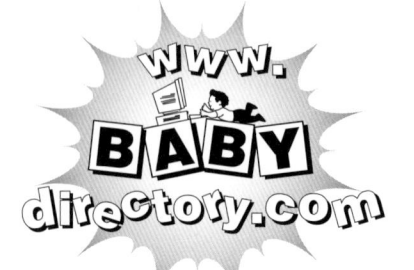

www.babydirectory.com The Local Baby Directory - *Surrey & S. Middlesex* **ORDER FORM**

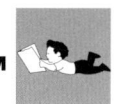

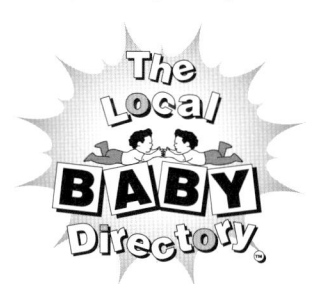

To order, call our Credit Card hotline on **020 8898 2411**
or order via our secure website at **www.babydirectory.com** *or* send this order form
with your payment to: **The Local Baby Directory: Surrey & S. Middlesex**
15 Lincoln Avenue, Twickenham, Middlesex TW2 6NH

Title	Price	Qty	Postage	Total
The Local Baby Directory				
Surrey & S. Middlesex (1-903288-09-6)	**£5.99**		**£1.00**	
Bristol, Bath & Somerset (1-903288-07-X)	£5.99		£1.00	
Herts & Middlesex (1-903288-08-8)	£5.99		£1.00	
Oxfordshire, Berks & Bucks (1-903288-02-9)	£4.99		£1.00	
South Wales (1-903288-06-1)	£4.99		£1.00	
Sussex & Hampshire (1-903288-05-3)	£4.99		£1.00	
The London Baby Directory (1-90328810-X)	£8.99		£1.50	
		Total Order Value		

Please print clearly

Name . . . .

Address . . . .

. . . .

. . . . Postcode . . . .

Tel . . . . E-mail address . . . .

METHOD OF PAYMENT *(please tick appropriate box)*

Cheque/Postal Order ☐   Credit Card ☐

Please make cheques payable to **The Local Baby Directory**

Card Number ☐☐☐☐ ☐☐☐☐ ☐☐☐☐ ☐☐☐☐ ☐☐☐☐

Issue No ☐☐   Expiry Date ☐☐☐☐   Valid from ☐☐☐☐

Signature . . . .

Code . . . .   If you do not wish to receive further information please tick ☐

FEEDBACK The Local Baby Directory - *Surrey & S. Middlesex* www.babydirectory.com

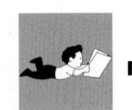

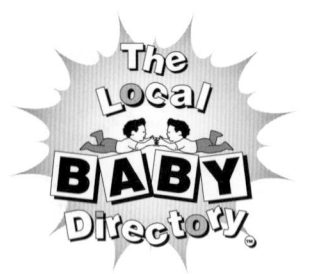

ADVERTISERS

If you provide a service or product we should know about, drop us a line, fax or e-mail. Listings are free, but we offer great advertising deals!

☐ This is a new product, service or facility.

☐ Please contact me with more information about advertising.

☐ Oops! You've missed this.

☐ Change of address, new branch, etc.

Category of product (eg, park, restaurant, nursery) ....

Name of product, service or facility ....

Address ....

....

Postcode .... Tel No ....

E-mail address .... www ....

Contact name and tel no *(if different from above)*

....

READERS

We would very much appreciate your comments. Errors, omissions, or poor service, please let us know. **A free copy of next year's book for the most useful comments!**

Feedback ....

....

....

....

Your own name, address, 'phone number, e-mail address (all optional)

....

....

Many thanks for taking the time to fill in this form
Please send completed form(s) to:

**The Local Baby Directory: Surrey & S. Middlesex,
15 Lincoln Avenue, Twickenham, Middlesex TW2 6NH
Tel: 020 8898 2411   E-mail: a_j_thompson@hotmail.com**

acupuncture

(see also complementary health)

Some recommend acupuncture in pregnancy for morning sickness and turning breech babies

British Acupuncture Council
63 Jeddo Road, W12. 020 8735 0400
Ring for list of practitioners

Cranleigh
David Reynolds
Smithbrook Clinic, 63a Smithbrook Kilns
01483 275500

Farnham
Oriental Medical Center
12, The Woolmead. 01252 718888

Guildford
Tim Foulsham
Vale End Chinese Health Clinic,
Chilworth Road, Albury. 01483 202556

Kingston-upon-Thames
Chinese Medicine Centre
64 Fife Road. 020 8546 3886

New Malden
Advanced Chinese Herbs & Acupuncture
156 High Street. 020 8949 2488

Old Oxted
Richard Cross
The Traditional Medical Centre,
2 Godstone Road. 01883 714036

Richmond
Dr Burn
Hermitage House, Church Terrace
020 8940 0164

Richmond Pharmacy Clinic
82-86 Sheen Road. 020 8940 3930

Sutton
Simon Bigwood
43 The Ridgeway. 020 8643 2599
www.acupuncture.co.uk

Wandsworth
Christine Hall
The Studio, 517 York Road. 020 8870 0566
Specialises in ante/post natal and children

Weybridge
Susan Sutton
Sturdie House, Broom Way. 01932 221268

adoption

Adoption UK
Manor Farm, Appletree Road, Chipping Warden, Banbury, Oxfordshire
01295 660121

British Agencies for Adoption and Fostering
Skyline House, 200 Union Street, London, SE1
020 7593 2060

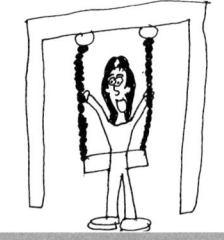

adventure playgrounds

(see also indoor adventure playcentres, parks & playgrounds)

These are usually for 5yrs and above.

Richmond
Richmond Adventure Playground
Behind Pools In the Park, Old Dear Park, Twickenham Road

Twickenham
Marble Hill Adventure Playground
Marble Hill Park, Richmond Road
Apr-Sep. Small charge. 5-15yrs

Visit us at
www.babydirectory.com

after school clubs

Many schools run after school clubs for their own and external pupils, usually from 3.30-6pm. Try your child's school, your local school, or ring the local Youth Service *(see councils)*

Kids' Club Network Helpline
020 7512 2100
www.kidsclubs.org.uk

Camberley
Tomlinscote Sports Centre
Tomlinscote Way, Frimley. 01276 670316
3yrs upwards

Feltham
Crane After School Hours
Crane Schools, Norman Avenue, Hanworth
020 8893 4450
4¹/₂ yrs upwards

Horley
Cranbrook (C.A.T.S Club)
Coppingham Cottage, Balcome Road
01293 823163
4-16yrs

Thornton Heath
Croydon Play Plus
020 8239 7189
Call for locations in Croydon area

alexander technique

(see also exercise classes, personal trainers)

Society of Teachers of the Alexander Technique
129 Camden Mews, NW1. 020 7284 3338

antenatal support & information

Information is available from your GP, your health clinic, the local maternity unit *(see hospitals)* and the organisations listed below

Active Birth Centre
25 Bickerton Road, London, N19
020 7482 5554

AIMS (Association for Improvement in Maternity Services)
5 Ann's Court, Grove Road, Surbiton
0870 765 1433
www.aims.org.uk

Independent Midwives' Association
1 The Great Quarry, Surrey. 01483 821104

National Childbirth Trust
Alexandra House, Oldham Terrace,
London, W3
Enquiry Line: 0870 444 8707

antenatal teachers

(see also antenatal support & information)

Antenatal teachers are often affiliated to the National Childbirth Trust or the Active Birth Centre. Maternity hospitals usually offer classes. Book early

Ruth Armes
020 8395 9435
Active birth teacher

Marjorie Dill
020 8948 5088

Kate Ingram
01932 863953
One-to-one classes

antenatal testing

Ask your GP or maternity unit for information. Most tests are available on the NHS

Antenatal Screening Service
020 7882 6293

Clinical Diagnostic Services
020 7483 3611/0099

Leeds Antenatal Screening Service
0113 234 4013

Ultrasound Diagnostic Services
020 7486 7991

arabic

Arabic School in Wimbledon
Wimbledon College, Edge Hill, London, SW19
01372 460 005
4-16yrs. Sats

aromatherapy

(see also baby toiletries, complementary health, massage)

International Federation of Aromatherapists
182 Chiswick High Road, London, W4
020 8742 2605
www.int-fed-aromatherapy.co.uk

mail order

Alpha Aromatherapy
01428 654421
Special blends available for pregnancy

AROMAKIDS
01278 671461
hippychick.ltd@virgin.net
www.hippychickproducts.com
Diverse range of essential-oil based toiletries for babies and toddlers

Beaming Baby
0800 0345 672

earth friendly baby
Healthquest Ltd, 7 Brampton Road, London, NW9. 020 8206 2066

Knots Elementals
020 8941 0759
mailorder@knotselementals.com
Also runs home learning sessions.
(A fun post-natal group activity!)

Natural Alternative
01531 650001

aromatherapists

Janine Healey
01737 550190

Sue Fortune
020 8332 9017

Coulsdon
Rosewell Natural Health Clinic
108a Brighton Road. 020 8763 2123

East Molesey
Essentials
12 Bridge Road. 020 8783 0371

Epsom
Gillian Tiplady Natural Therapies
30a The Parade. 01372 722185

New Malden
Natural Woman Health & Beauty Clinic
82a High Street. 020 8336 0366

Redhill
Nicola Fry Health & Beauty Centre
1 Hatchlands Road. 01737 765640

Ruth Hersey
Ponds Corner, 13 Spencer Way, Earlswood
01737 773497
Will visit you at home

Reigate
Jakki Todd
53a Lesbourne Road. 01737 223788

Richmond
Richmond Pharmacy Clinic
82-86 Sheen Road. 020 8940 3930

Sutton
Aromatherapy at the Dolphin Room
142 St James Road. 020 8642 6519

Twickenham
Essential Therapies
020 8892 8538

Lesley Corbet
020 8255 9666

Visit us at
www.babydirectory.com

aromatherapy (cont.)

Walton-on-Thames
Sally Ann Rees
Lifestyle Natural Health Centre,
4 The Shopping Centre, Hersham Green
01932 254624

Woking
Bourne Health
Bourne House, Horsell Park. 01483 722122

art

(see also ceramics, dance, drama, music)

Art for Tots
01372 386520

Brentford
Watermans Art Centre
40 High Street. 020 8232 1020
Completely refurbished

Kew
Crafty Kids
020 8241 7660
After school club for 5-11yrs. Classes in Kew & Barnes

astrological charts

Astrological Baby Profiles
32 High Street, Scotter, Lincs, DN21 3TW
01724 761404

ChildStar
01473 240276

au pair agencies

(see also babysitters, childminders, nanny agencies)

Au pairs live-in and help with housework, childcare and babysitting. They are not generally recommended for very small babies

AU PAIR INTERNATIONAL
118 Cromwell Road, London SW7
020 7370 3798
www.apni.org.uk

FRIENDS AU PAIR AGENCY
020 8847 0920/07789 646730
www.friendsaupairs.com

HOME AWAY FROM HOME
020 8763 1206
www.homeawayfromhomechildcare.co.uk

JOLAINE AU PAIR AGENCY
020 8449 1334

LARAH AU-PAIRS
01932 341704

MONTROSE AGENCY INTERNATIONAL
23 Bullescroft Road, Edgware,
Middx, HA8 8RN
020 8958 9209
montrose@taylor.clara.net
We listen, we care, we make the right connections. Established 22 years
See advert under nanny agencies

RICHMOND & TWICKENHAM AU PAIRS & NANNIES
01283 716611
vicki@rtaupairs.demon.co.uk
www.aupairsnationwide.co.uk
Established in 1992. Friendly efficient service. French, Spanish, Italian, Czech and Slovak

FRIENDS Au Pair Agency
European Au Pair Specialist
020 8847 0920
friendsaupairs@mailcity.com
www.friendsaupairs.com

Au Pair / Nanny NETWORK INTERNATIONAL
118 Cromwell Road, SW7 4ET
Tel: 020 7370 3798   Fax: 020 7370 4718

The Childcare People
who care for your family
Au Pairs, Mother's Help and Nannies carefully screened and personally interviewed available all year around.

Continental Nannies
Looking for a Nanny from France, Scandinavia or from another European Country? We specialise in Continental Nannies to bring a little je ne sais quoi to your family.

Why choose us?
You owe it to your family to work with the agency that will provide you with the best quality service, most rigorously selected childcarers and the peace of mind that comes with a customer care guarantee.

APPLY ON LINE
from May 2002 @ www.apni.org.uk
or email: sandrine@apni.org.uk

Founder Member International Au Pair Association

Larah Au-Pairs
Au-Pairs available now, long term & summer placements to help with your childcare needs and general housework.
All our Au-Pairs are carefully selected and we offer personal friendly service
Tel: 01932 341704
E mail larahaupairs@nationwideisp.net

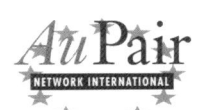

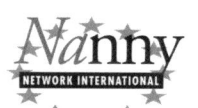

RICHMOND AND TWICKENHAM
Au Pairs & Nannies
Vicki Whitwell
The Old Parsonage, 15-17 Main Street,
Barton under Needham, Staffordshire DE13 8AA
Tel: 01283 716611
Fax: 01283 712299
email: vicki@rtaupairs.demon.co.uk
www.aupairsnationwide.co.uk
Mobile: 0780 1710967

HOME Away From HOME
International Childcare

- ❖ **Au Pairs**
- ❖ **Nannies**
- ❖ **Parents' Help**
- ❖ **After school pickup/care**
- ❖ **Babysitters**
- ❖ **Domestics**

All carers have references and are fully vetted
Au pairs available from most
EC/non-EC countries
(National coverage)
For your Childcare Needs Call:

Tel: 020 8763 1206
Fax: 020 8405 0678
Mobile: 07764 341777

Email: homeawayfromhome@bigfoot.com
www.homeawayfromhomechildcare.co.uk

---

www.BABYdirectory.com
Advice On-Line

Wanted Baby Scientists!

We are recruiting babies (Birth-12 mo.) to take part in fun studies at our Babylab. We provide a black cab service if you live within 5 miles of our Centre, or we will refund your travel expenses. If you would like to discover how babies learn, please contact Jane at the Babylab.

The Babylab, Birkbeck College
32 Torrington Sq., London WC1E 7JL
Tel: 020 7631 6258
email: babylab@bbk.ac.uk, www.psyc.bbk.ac.uk

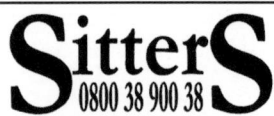

Sitters
0800 38 900 38

For Evening Babysitters
www.sitters.co.uk
Evening Babysitters with Professional Childcare Experience
0800 38 900 38
www.sitters.co.uk
Please quote ref: Baby Directory

baby research

BABYLAB
Centre for Brain & Cognitive Development, FREEPOST,
32 Torrington Square, WC1E 7JL
020 7631 6258
Have fun with your baby making discoveries about the brain

baby toiletries

Beaming Baby
0800 0345 672

earth friendly baby
Healthquest Ltd, 7 Brampton Road,
London, NW9 9BX. 020 8206 2066

Green People
01444 410444
info@greenpeople.co.uk

Dr Hauschka
01386 792622
Natural sun creams for children
(+ great adult skincare range!)

Guildford
Neal's Yard Remedies
2 Market Street. 01483 450434

Richmond
Neal's Yard Remedies
15 King Street. 020 8948 9248

babysitters

(see also childminders, nanny agencies)

SITTERS
0800 38 900 38
www.sitters.co.uk
SITTERS - the UK's leading and ONLY national evening babysitting service

Childminders
6 Nottingham Street, London, W1
020 7935 3000

Cranleigh
Kiddikare Babysitting Service for Surrey
9 Thurlow Walk. 01483 271241
www.kiddikareuk.co.uk

Esher
Mary Ward
The Cottage, 74 Lower Green Road
01372 469552
Mother/ex-maternity nurse will babysit your new born

Twickenham
Motherstime
5th Floor Regal House, London Road
020 8892 9293

The Richmond Childminding Group
55 Heath Road. 020 8891 6090

Woking
Abbies Aunties
16 Abbey Road, Horsell. 01483 772214

Visit us at
www.babydirectory.com

benefits

Benefits Agency
Department of Social Security,
CBC Washington, Newcastle-upon-Tyne,
NE88 1AA. 08701 555501

Maternity Alliance
45 Beech Street, Barbican, London, EC2Y 8AD
020 7588 8582
Advice on benefits, maternity rights at work

birth announcements

(see also cards)

Announce It
01306 628116

CHATTERBOX CARDS
PO Box 142, Beckenham, Kent, BR3 6ZL
020 8650 8650
www.chatterboxcards.com
Personalised birth announcements and christening invitations. Delivered in 3 days. Free brochure

HAPPY HANDS
7 Brockwell Park Row, Tulse Hill,
London SW2. 020 8671 2020
info@happyhands.ws
www.happyhands.ws

Hyper Bubba
contact@hyperbubba.com
www.hyperbubba.com
Hyper Bubba creates funky, unusual and personalised birth announcement websites

Printed Birth Announcements and Party Invitations
Unit 5, Philpotts Yard, Beare Green, Dorking
01306 713630
www.printed4u.co.uk

Tots Pots
020 8979 4176 / 07903 187690
Have your newborns foot or handprint glazed onto a plate

Personalised Birth Announcements & Christening Invitations

- Distinctive and fun designs
- Quick - posted to you in 3 days
- Prices from £32.00 for 25 inc p&p

For your FREE Chatterbox Cards brochure
Telephone **020 8650 8650**
www.chatterboxcards.com
• birth announcements • party invitations
• change of address cards
• announcements for all occasions

You're Amazing !
Now tell the World your news

Birth Announcement Cards
with
Your own baby's footprints
(inkless print kit provided)

Call **HappyHands** on
020 8671 2020

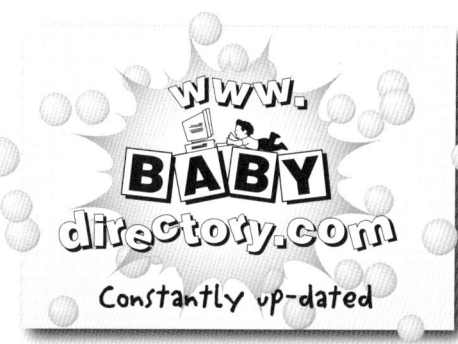

---

www.BABYdirectory.com
Constantly up-dated

Please say you saw the ad in
The Local Baby Directory

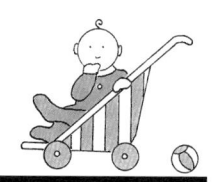

Celebrate Your Pregnancy

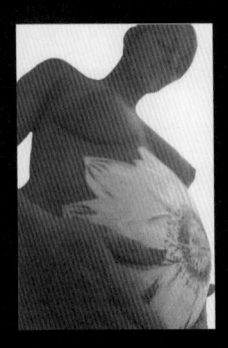

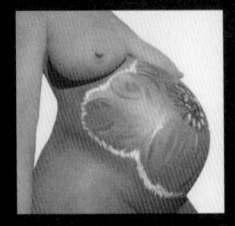

Body Painting for Pregnant Women

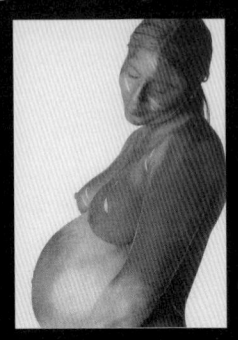

Become a canvas for the day and remember your pregnancy forever
For more information contact:

Julia Laderman

07803 121923   www.embody.org.uk   info@embody.org.uk

body painter

Body Painting for Pregnant Women
07803 121923
www.embody.org.uk
Become a canvas for the day and remember your pregnancy forever

book clubs for children

Letterbox Library
71-73 Allan Road, London, N16 8RY
020 7503 4801

Red House Books Ltd
The Red House, Windrush Park, Witney, Oxford, OX29 0YD. 01993 893472

book shops for children

Major chains such as Books etc, Hammicks, W. H. Smith, Waterstone's have good children's sections. Visit our website at www.babydirectory.com for a selection of the best children's books

Banstead
Ibis Bookshop
109 High Street. 01737 353260

Camberley
Ottakars
6-8 Grace Reynolds Walk, Main Square
01276 65227

Caterham
Titles of Caterham
32 Church Walk Shopping Centre
01883 347196

Cobham
Methven's Booksellers
12a Anyards Road. 01932 862903

Please say you saw the ad in
The Local Baby Directory

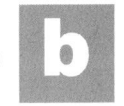

Coulsdon
Turners Bookshop
46 Chipstead Valley Road. 020 8660 1432

Cranleigh
The Book Shop
123 High Street. 01483 274265

Crawley
Ottakars
Units 4-6,The Martleys. 01293 525352

Croydon
The Works
143 North End. 020 8760 0558

Waterstone's
1063-7 Whitgift Centre. 020 8686 7032

Dorking
Waterstone's
54-60 South Street. 01306 886884

Epsom
Hammicks Bookshops
18 The Ashley Centre. 01372 742533

Farnham
Hammicks Bookshops
11 Lion & Lamb Yard. 01252 724666

Godalming
The Surrey Bookshop
59 High Street. 01483 420888

Guildford
Thomas Thorpe's
170 High Street. 01483 562770

Waterstone's
35-39 North Street. 01483 302919

Waterstone's
50-54 High Street. 01483 457545

Haslemere
Haslemere Bookshop
2 Causeway Side, High Street. 01428 652952

Hindhead
Grayshott Books
8 The Square, Grayshott. 01428 604798

Horley
Horley Bookshop
22 High Street. 01293 783558

Smallfield Books & Gifts
1 Wheelers Lane, Smallfield. 01342 842001

Kew
Kew Bookshop
1-2 Station Approach. 020 8940 0030

Kingston-upon-Thames
Borders
Unit 1, Charter Key, Market Place
020 8974 9444

Waterstone's
23-25 Thames Street. 020 8547 1221

Waterstone's
Unit S9, Wood Street, The Bentalls Centre
020 8974 6811

Redhill
Hammicks Bookshops
12-13 The Belfry Centre. 01737 770334

Richmond
The Lion & Unicorn Bookshop
19 King Street. 020 8940 0483

The Open Book
10 King Street. 020 8940 1802

Piccolo Bella
6 Eton Street. 020 8948 8601
thetoy-station.com

Waterstone's
2-6 Hill Street. 020 8332 1600

Staines
Ottakars
77 High Street. 01784 490404

Surbiton
Regency Bookshops
45 Victoria Road. 020 8399 2188

Sutton
Baines Bookshop
3 Lower Square Civic Centre, St Nicholas Way
020 8661 1677

Kendrake Children's Bookshop
216 St Nicholas Centre. 020 8255 7744

Waterstone's
71-81 High Street. 020 8770 0404

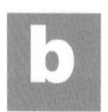

book shops for children (cont.)

Teddington
Broad Street Books
43a Broad Street. 020 8614 5777

Teddington Book Shop
55 High Street. 020 8977 4301

Twickenham
The Bookstore
19 King Street. 020 8744 3030

Langton's Bookshop
44-45 Church Street. 020 8892 3800

Walton-on-Thames
The Bookstore
44 High Street. 01932 254455

Weybridge
Weybridge Books
28 Church Street. 01932 842498

Woking
Hammicks Bookshops
16-18 Wolsey Walk. 01483 726938

James Thin Ltd
Unit 44, The Peacocks Centre. 01483 766756

Methven's Booksellers
Surrey House, 46 Commercial Way
01483 771407

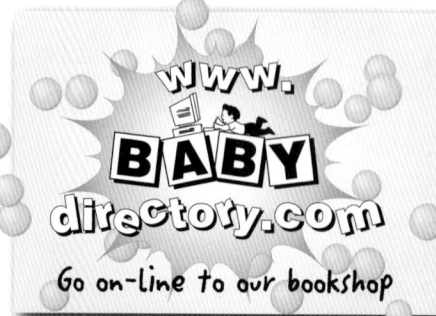

breastfeeding

advice

Visit our website at www.babydirectory.com for e-mail advice and information from National Childbirth Trust and Breastfeeding Network counsellors

Breastfeeding Network
0870 900 8787

Association of Breastfeeding Mothers
PO Box 207, Bridgewater, Somerset, TA6 7YT
020 7813 1481
24hr volunteer counselling service

La Leche League
BM Box 3424, London, WC1N 3XX
020 7242 1278
24hr counselling service. Local groups have monthly meetings

National Childbirth Trust Breastfeeding Counsellors
0870 444 8708

accessories

Ameda Egnell Ltd
Unit1, Belvedere Trading Estate, Taunton
01823 336362
Breast pump hire.

Baby Bliss
020 8568 4914

Bussom Buddies
42b Colwell Road, East Dulwich
020 8516 3212

Expressions Breastfeeding
CMS House, Basford House, Leek
01538 386650

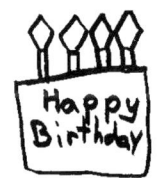

cakes

(see also party catering)

Coughlans Pattisserie
020 8684 2304
Call for locations throughout Surrey

Too Nice To Slice
020 8892 9013

Camberley
Carly's Cake Box
301 London Road. 01276 692514

Carshalton
Nozzles Cake Craft
103 Streetanley Park Road. 020 8669 8566
Cake decorations

Chiddingfold
Roney's Cakes of Quality
Low Prestwick Cottage, Prestwick Lane
01428 652924

East Molesey
Blue Ribbons
110 Walton Road. 020 8941 1591

Epsom
Corteil & Barratt
40 High Street, Ewell Village. 020 8393 0032

Farnham
Squire's Kitchens
Alfred House, Holmes Business Park,
3 Waverley Lane. 01252 711749
Cake decorations

Leatherhead
Cascade Too
19 High Street, Gt Bookham. 01372 450105

New Malden
Nikki Brown
020 8336 0395

Redhill
Cakes for Occasions
Cherry Tree House, 25 Park View Road,
Salfords. 01293 409460

Richmond
Kookes Unlimited
16 Eton Street. 020 8940 8448
Cake accessories

Surbiton
Blackburn's Cake Accessories Centre
108 Alexandra Drive. 020 8399 6875

Woking
Dial-a-Cake
01483 769786

Speciality Cakes
9 High Street, Knaphill. 01483 797610

car seats & accessories

(see also nursery goods)

Baby's First Wave
www.babysfirstwave.com
The first drive home car flag

Motor Hoods
0800 163725
www.motorhoods.co.uk
Turns an estate car into a 7 seater

cards

(see also birth announcements)

CHATTERBOX CARDS
PO Box 142, Beckenham, Kent, BR3 6ZL
020 8650 8650
www.chatterboxcards.com
Personalised birth announcements and christening invitations. Delivered in 3 days. Free brochure
See advert under birth announcements

Announce It
01306 628116

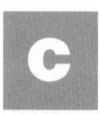

carriers

CHILD HIP SEAT
Hippychick Ltd, Barford Gables,
Spaxton, Bridgwater,
Somerset, TA5 1AE
01278 671461
hippychick.ltd@virgin.net
www.hippychickproducts.com
Innovative back-supporting belt with integral seat for carrying children (6mths-3yrs). Endorsed by osteopaths

Better Baby Sling
01923 444442
www.betterbabysling.co.uk
"Wonderfully easy to put on – very comfortable" The Independent

Huggababy Natural Baby Products
19-21 The Prya Centre, Talgarth, Brecon, Powys. 01874 711629

Wilkinet
PO Box 20, Cardigan, SA43 1JB. 0800 138 3400

cassettes & CDs

Move and Groove with Paint Pots
020 7376 4571
32 songs for all ages

Cover to Cover Cassettes
PO Box 112, Marlborough,
Wiltshire, SN8 3UG. 01672 562255

castings

Casts, usually of hands or feet, preserved in bronze, glass or on ceramic tiles

GOLDEN HANDS, SILVER FEET LTD.
Unit G. Homesdale Centre,
216-218 Homesdale Road,
Bromley, Kent BR1 2QZ
www.goldenhands.co.uk

Happy Hands
7 Brockwell Park Row, Tulse Hill, London, SW2 2YH. 020 8671 2020
info@happyhands.ws
www.happyhands.ws
Hand and foot prints and works of art preserved on ceramic tiles

cerebral palsy

Centre for Children with Cerebral Palsy
54 Muswell Hill, N10. 020 8444 7242
The Hornsey Trust runs a conductive education centre

ceramics

Immortalise baby's footprint on a plate! Also a good venue for older children's parties.

Ashtead
PaintPots
Marsden Garden Centre, Pleasure Pit Road
01372 273891

Claygate
Brush and Bisque-it
7 The Parade. 01372 462447

Farnham
Ceramics Café
44c Frensham Road, Lower Bourne
01252 821021

Kew
Crafty Kids
020 8241 7660
After school club for 5-11yrs
Classes in Kew & Barnes

The Ceramics Café
1a Mortlake Terrace. 020 8332 6661

Kingston-upon-Thames
Brush and Bisque-It
4 Eden Street. 020 8546 3393

Ripley
Ceramics Café
High Street. 01483 224477

Sutton
VILLAGE CERAMICS
31 Station Way, Cheam Village
020 8661 7837
www.villageceramics.co.uk
Regular classes, Kids club on Saturday, Birthday parties, group sessions. Footprints forever - create a ceramic or plate from your childs foot or hand print.

Twickenham
Pottery Café
332 Richmond Road. 020 8744 3000

Weybridge
Dynamic Ceramic
49 Church Street. 01932 846782

chemists: late opening

In case of emergency, police stations should have information on local chemists which may stay open late

chess

Richmond Junior Chess Club
020 8898 0362
6yrs+

childcare listing magazine

SIMPLY CHILDCARE
16 Bushey Hill Road, London, SE5
020 7701 6111
www.simplychildcare.com

Please say you saw the ad in
The Local Baby Directory

Footprints Forever

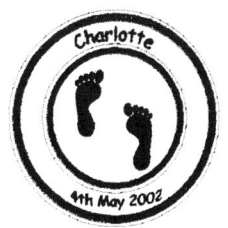

Capture an everlasting memory of your young one's early years
Your child's foot or handprints imortalised in ceramics
A wide range of plates & mugs from £20
Arrange a Footprints Forever party in your own home or visit our studio
Call for a brochure or appointment

Village Ceramics
31 Station Way · Cheam Village · Sutton
020 8661 7837

Need a Nanny? Childminder? Nannyshare? Au Pair? Mother's Help? Don't know where to look? Don't know what to do? Then try

Simply Childcare
the childcare listings magazine

It has lots of people offering childcare & lots of parents looking for childcare: part-time, full-time, temporary, occasional. Read Simply Childcare & solve your problem. For details call

020 7701 6111
website: www.simplychildcare.com
email: info@simplychildcare.com

PLUS if you need unbiased, up-to-date, practical information on all aspects of finding and handling childcare e.g. different kinds of childcare, their merits & drawbacks, costs, tax/NIC, interviewing, contracts, police checks, etc then send a cheque for our Childcare Information Pack (£9.95) to Simply Childcare, 16 Bushey Hill Road, London SE5 8QJ

As recommended in local & national press

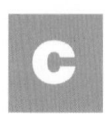

childminders

(see also au pair agencies, babysitters, nanny agencies)

For lists of registered childminders in your area, contact your local social services department *(see councils)*

Childcare Link
www.childcarelink.gov.uk

Children's Information Service
Free information and advice on childcare, at Mothercare World, Kew Retail Park. Tues 12.30-2pm. 020 8831 6298

www.childminders.co.uk
020 7487 4578

National Childminding Association
020 8464 6164

Surrey Chlidren's Information Service
www.surreycc.gov.uk/earlyyearsandchildcare

Croydon
Croydon Childminding Association
Cornerstone House, 14 Willis Road
020 8683 2105

Isleworth
Marlborough Minders
Marlborough School, London Road
020 8560 9299

chiropractic

Suitable for treating back and neck pain. May be useful for colic in babies

British Chiropractic Association
0118 950 5950

McTimoney Chiropractic Association
21 High Street, Eynsham, Oxfordshire
01865 880974

Back to Health Chiropractic Clinics
020 8546 6880
Various locations

christening gowns

CHRISTENING GOWNS
35 Derwent Crescent, Kettering, Northamptonshire
01536 515401
julie@christeningoutfits.co.uk
www.christeningoutfits.co.uk
Over four hundred gowns and rompersuits in stock, plus accessories

JAC & BETY
14 Church Street, Twickenham
020 8892 3776
See advert under nursery goods

Little Angels
15 The Market, Wrythe Lane, Rose Hill, Carshalton. 020 8641 0687

Thimbelina
7 Acremead Road, Wheatley, Oxfordshire
01865 872549
Hand-smocked heirloom gowns, outfits and accessories handmade to order

cinemas

Many cinemas have a Saturday morning junior screening

cleaners

SELCLENE
01932 567649

clinics

Staffed by health visitors and community doctors, clinics provide health and development checks and are a good source of information and supplementary health care (e.g. family planning, chiropody, eye checks)

SELCLENE

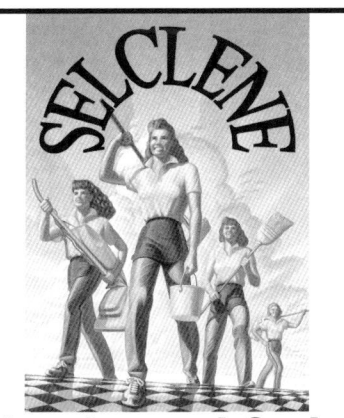

Cleaning and Caring for your Home

Serving: Richmond, Twickenham, Teddington, Hampton and surrounding areas. Established, high quality cleaning & ironing service provided by experienced & reliable cleaners. Fully Insured.

Call 01639 730 205
Fax: 01639 731077 Email: yacomine@aol.com
www.selclene.co.uk

clothing shops

(see also mail order, maternity wear, nearly new shops, nursery goods, shoe shops)

We have not listed the major chains, eg. Adams, Baby Gap, Boots, Hennes, Jigsaw Junior, John Lewis, Marks & Spencer, Monsoon, Mothercare, Next, etc which can be found in most high streets

Janalli Children's Clothes Parties
07788 636827

Addlestone
Pixies
5 The Broadway, New Haw
01932 349864

Ashford
Madhatters
62 Church Road. 01784 253187

Dorking
Flapjacks
St Martins Walk Shopping Centre
01306 743320
www.flapjacks.org.uk

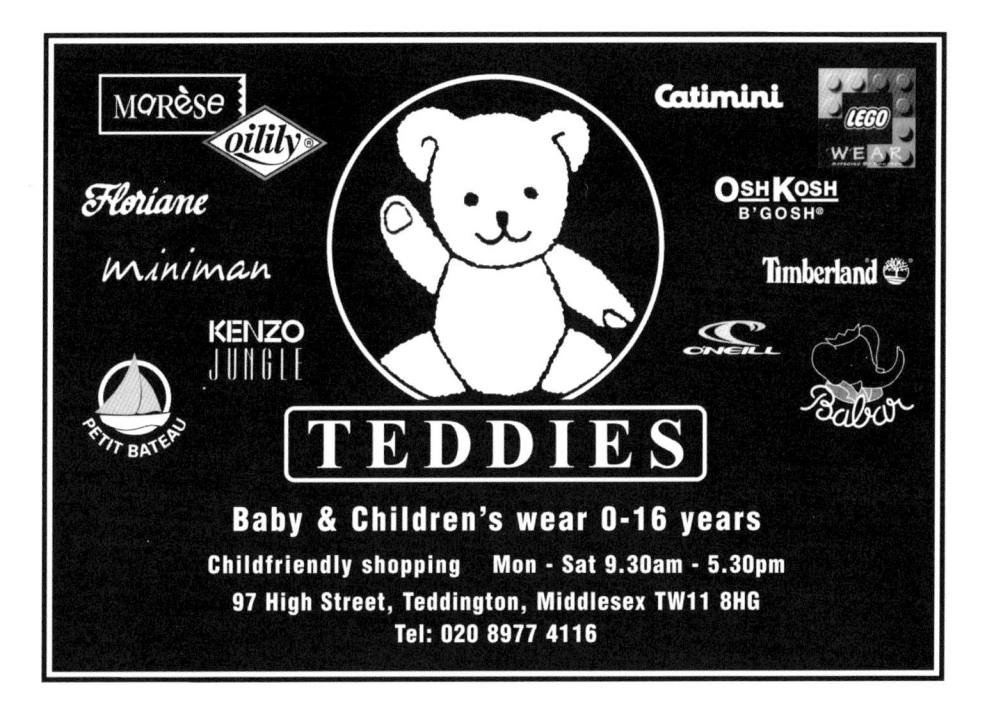

TEDDIES

Morèse · Oilily · Floriane · Miniman · Kenzo Jungle · Petit Bateau · Catimini · Lego Wear · OshKosh B'Gosh · Timberland · O'Neill · Babar

Baby & Children's wear 0-16 years
Childfriendly shopping   Mon - Sat 9.30am - 5.30pm
97 High Street, Teddington, Middlesex TW11 8HG
Tel: 020 8977 4116

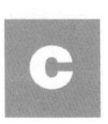

clothing shops (cont.)

East Molesey
Little Monkey
91 Walton Road. 020 8941 1255

Esher
Magic Roundabout
16 The Parade, Claygate. 01372 467984

Ewell Village
Freeways
77 High Street. 020 8393 0078

Guildford
Gymboree
71 High Street. 01483 303308

Hedgehog
12 Chertsey Street. 01483 575088

Haslemere
Footprints
rear of 34 High Street. 01428 643676
0-13yrs

Kingston-upon-Thames
Catimini
38 High Street. 020 8541 4635

Leatherhead
Over The Moon
25 High Street, Great Bookham. 01372 452509
0-8yrs

Oxted
JJ's Childrenswear
36 Station Road West. 01883 715262
0-16yrs

Reigate
Baby Days
84 High Street. 01737 241126
www.babydays-e.com

Richmond
Gymboree
53 George Street. 020 8940 9350
2-10yrs

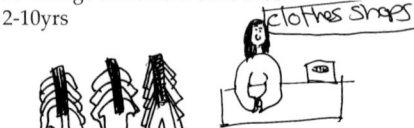

PICCOLO BELLA
6 Eton Street. 020 8948 8601
thetoy-station.com
Children's wear 0-6yrs. Dressing up clothes and accessories. Toys and books

Teddington
TEDDIES
97 High Street. 020 8977 4116
See advert on page 15

Twickenham
Happicraft
46-48 London Road. 020 892 5262

JAC & BETY
14 Church Street, Twickenham
020 8892 3776
See advert under nursery goods

Weybridge
Red Balloon
32 Baker Street. 01932 844 065

clubs

Scouts Association
Bury Road, E4. 0845 300 1818
Beaver Scouts 6-8yrs. Cubs 8-10yrs

Girl Guiding UK
17-19 Buckingham Palace Road, SW1
020 7834 6242
Rainbow Guides 5-7yrs. Brownies 7-10yrs

complementary health

(see also acupuncture, aromatherapy, homeopathy, massage, osteopathy, reflexology, yoga)

Association of Systemic Kinesiology
020 8399 3215

Complementary Medicine Association (CMA)
020 8305 9571

Institute for Complementary Medicine
PO Box 194, London, SE16 1QZ
Send sae for list of local addresses

Little Miracles
PO Box 3896, London, NW3 7DS
020 7431 6153
Flower essences - gentle remedies

National Institute of Medical Herbalists
01392 426022

ALOE VERA HEALTH & BEAUTY
020 8608 1857
kateandchris@blueyonder.co.uk
See advert under natural products

Beauty at Home
020 8743 8579

THE KEEPER
020 8608 1857
kateandchris@blueyonder.co.uk
Reusable sanitary protection. Unique product, environmental, convenient, economical. 90 day money-back guarantee

Camberley
Camberley Natural Therapy Centre
9 Tekels Park. 01276 23300
sue@kalicinska.freeserve.co.uk

East Molesey
MARTINE L.FAURE-ALDERSON HEALTH CLINIC
187 Ember Lane. 020 8398 6943

Hampton
Nicky Wesson
26 Church Street. 020 8941 6652
Medical herbalist. Treasure trove of ante/post natal and children's natural products!

Richmond
Richmond Pharmacy Clinic
82-86 Sheen Road. 020 8940 3930

Twickenham
Maple Leaf Clinic
20 The Green. 020 8255 9266
Call for list of therapies. Good source of complementary health products

Woking
Bourne Health
Bourne House, Horsell Park. 01483 722122

The Clinic of Natural Therapies

Gentle treatments for babies and all the family
We offer a wide variety of complementary therapies including cranial osteopathy, homeopathy and acupuncture.

187 Ember Lane, East Molesey, Surrey KT8 OBU
020 8398 6943

---

computers for children

Interactive Kids
020 8891 1644
alayne@interactive-kids.co.uk

Thames Ditton
Computer Gym Software School
The Courtyard, 27a High Street. 020 8224 6444
4-14yrs

concerts

Barbican
Silk Street, London EC2. 020 7638 8891
LSO Family Concerts

English Heritage Musical Summer Evenings
020 7973 3427
Concerts at Kenwood, Marble Hill House

cookery

Dodo Cookbook
PO Box 10507, London, N22 7WZ
0870 900 8004
www.dodopad.com

Fun Food Academy
01243 573975
Cookery classes during termtime (and cookery workshops in the holidays) for 4-11yrs. Also children's cookery birthday parties. Godalming area

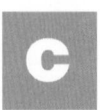

councils

Your local council is an excellent source of information. Ask for the Under 8s section, Early Years' section, or leisure. They can provide lists of local nurseries, schools, parks, etc. Some produce excellent booklets on their area.

Elmbridge Borough Council
01372 474474

Epsom & Ewell Borough Council
01372 732000

Guildford Borough Council
01483 505050

Hounslow Borough Council
020 8583 2000
www.hounslow.gov.uk
A-Z Guide for 0-12s

Kingston-upon-Thames Borough Council
020 8547 6582
www.rbkc.gov.uk
Children's Information Service

Merton Borough Council
020 8543 2222

Mole Valley District Council
01306 885001

Reigate & Banstead Borough Council
01737 276000

Richmond Borough Council
020 8891 1411
www.richmond.gov.uk

Runnymede Borough Council
01932 838383

Spelthorne Borough Council
01784 451499

Surrey Heath Borough Council
01276 686152

Tandridge Borough Council
01883 722000

Waverley Borough Council
01483 755855

Woking Borough Council
01483 755855

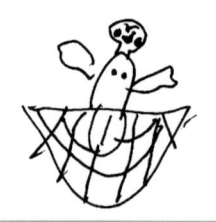

cradles

(see also nursery furniture & décor)

Swingers & Rockers
Terfyn Uchaf, Rhiw, Pwllheli, Gwyned
01758 780305
www.cradles.co.uk

craniosacral therapy

(see also osteopathy)

Craniosacral Therapy Association
07000 784735

Twickenham
Lesley Corbet
020 8255 9666

crèches: mobile

The Mobile Crèche Co.
01423 797440

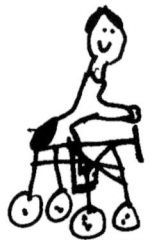

cycling & cycling attachments

Christiania Tricycle
Zero Emissions 020 7723 2409
Family trailers

Parks, Playgrounds and Pubs
020 8946 0912

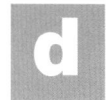

dance

(see also art, drama, gym, music)

Dance teachers tend to hold classes in different halls within a general area, so check neighbouring areas, as the teacher may be listed there. Most ballet classes are for children from 3 years upwards unless otherwise stated.

Royal Academy of Dancing
020 7326 8000
Can provide lists. From 3yrs

Imperial Society of Teachers of Dancing
020 7377 1577
Contact for list, specifying which type of dance for 5yrs+

International Dance Teachers' Association Ltd
Ring for a list of teachers in your area

Chessington
Genesis Dance Works
01372 742517
Chessington & Epsom. 2^1/$_2$ yrs+

Ewell Village
Dance to Enjoy
020 8399 1596
3-11yrs, Sat. mornings

Feltham
Georgina's Dance School
74 Hampton Lane, Hanworth. 020 8755 1504

Kington-upon-Thames
Kingston Ballet School
020 8549 1129

Kingston Vale Dance Academy
St John's Church Hall, Robin Hood Roundabout. 020 8579 4652
4yrs+

Leatherhead
Linkside Studios For Dance
01372 378398
From 2^1/$_2$yrs. Classes in Caterham & Leatherhead

Staines
Jeanne Bamforth School of Dancing
01784 241369

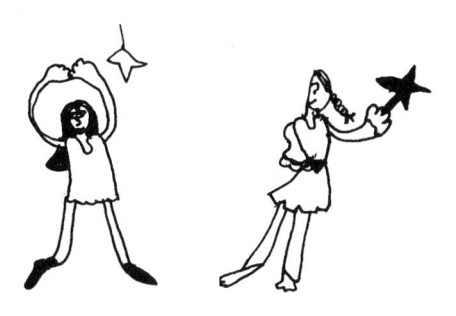

Parry School of Dancing
01784 453390

Tolworth
Gina Van Dyke Stage School
The Studios, Fairmead. 020 8399 9429

Twickenham
Danceforce School of Dancing
55 Manor Court, Manor Road. 020 8894 7306

Geraldine Maguire
020 8892 3006
Ballet from 3yrs

London Dance School
020 8940 3793
Chiswick & Twickenham

Wallington
Willow School of Dance
020 8398 6532
From 2^1/$_2$yrs. Wallington, Purley & Tolworth

dentists

British Homeopathic Association
27a Devonshire Street, London. 020 7566 7800
Call for a list of homeopathic dentists

Wonersh Dental Centre
3-4 The Common, Wonersh. 01483 898427
Holistic dental practice

Visit us at
www.babydirectory.com

01795 428150
sioux.lbgraphics@blueyonder.co.uk
complete creative solutions
small business specialists

lb graphics — design & print

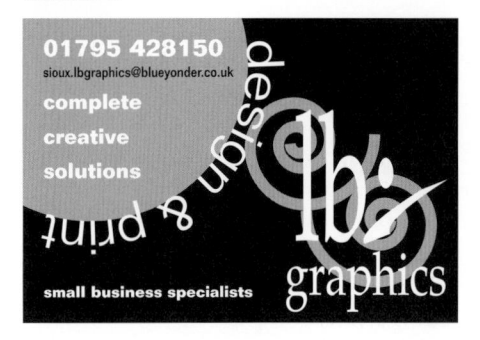

designers

LB Graphics
01795 428150
sioux.lbgraphics@blueyonder.co.uk
Small business specialists

designer outlets

Ashford Designer Outlet
Ashford, Kent. 01223 895900
Junction 10, M20. Signposted

Bicester Village
Bicester, Oxfordshire. 01869 323200

Great Western Designer Outlet
Kemble Drive, Swindon. 01793 507600
Junction 16, M4

dolls' houses

(see also toy shops)

Dorking
Dolls House Gallery
23 West Street. 01306 885785

Epsom
The Copper Kettle
6 East Street. 01372 722221

Guildford
The Bear Garden & Dolls Attic
10 Jeffries Passage. 01483 302581

Shepperton
Small Talk
96 High Street. 01932 247686

Sunbury-on-Thames
Fantazia Dolls
01932 780934
Doll maker

Sutton
The Dolls House
122 St Nicholas Centre, St Nicholas Way
020 8401 0170
Collectible dolls plus dolls houses

West Byfleet
Through The Keyhole
25-26 Station Approach. 01932 355571

Worcester Park
Dolly's Dolls House & Miniatures
19 Cheam Common Road. 020 8337 5663

doulas

A doula provides physical, emotional and practical support for the family during pregnancy, labour and immediately after the birth. The area mentioned is where the doula is based. They will normally travel to a much wider area

Doula UK
PO Box 33187, London, N8 9AW
www.doula.org.uk

www.britishdoulas.co.uk

Cheam
Tinies Nanny Agency
020 8642 2228
n.surrey@tinieschildcare.co.uk
www.tinieschildcare.co.uk

Croydon
Hefferlumps & Co.
07803 589171
heffperlumpsandco@another.com

Dorking
Fairygodmother Doulas
01306 711581 / 01306 712582
www.fairygodmotherdoulas.co.uk

Hilary Lewin
01306 730793

Farnborough
Tinies Nanny Agency
01252 371373
hants@tinieschildcare.co.uk
www.tinieschildcare.co.uk

Fulham
Maggie Vaughan
020 7731 5096
North West Surrey area

Guildford
Louise Warmerdam
01483 450691

Merstham
Tinies Nanny Agency
01737 642444
e.surrey@tinieschildcare.co.uk
www.tinieschildcare.co.uk

Shepperton
Penny Bradley
01932 782046

Teddington
Ruth Hayman
020 8977 4394

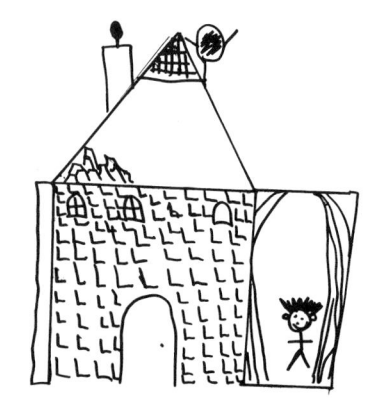

drama

(see also art, dance, gym, music and theatres which often run drama courses)

Julia Gabriel Speech & Drama Centre
020 8405 3222
Classes in Twickenham, Kingston, Sutton, Purley & Kingston Vale
4-16yrs

Perform Schools
020 7209 3805
Richmond & Kingston
4-7yrs

Cobham
The Cat's Grin
53 Oxshott Way. 01932 867698
4-11yrs

Croydon
Helen O'Grady Drama Academy
020 8662 0962
5yrs+

Esher
Chadsworth Stage School
21 Hinchley Drive, Hinchley Wood
020 8398 8104
2-18yrs

Kingston-upon-Thames
Helen O'Grady Drama Academy
020 8894 0804
5yrs+

Reigate
Italia Conti Associate School
Dunnotar School, High Trees Road
020 8644 9317

Walton-on-Thames
Stagecoach Theatre Arts School
The Courthouse, Elm Grove. 01932 254333
Acting, singing and dancing

Visit us at
www.babydirectory.com

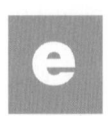

educational consultants

(see also helplines: education, schools, tuition)

GABBITAS EDUCATIONAL CONSULTANTS
Carrington House,
126-130 Regent Street, London, W1
020 7734 0161
admin@gabbitas.co.uk
www.gabbitas.com
See advert under schools

ISCis London and South East
35-37 Grosvenor Gardens, London, SW1
020 7798 1560
Free handbook listing all accredited independent schools

Society of Childhood Education
LBS Forum, 97 Cornwell Road,
London, SW7. 020 020 7581 9357
A support and information society for parents/guardians and nannies/au pairs; members also include teachers, educational experts

exercise for ante- and post-natal

(see also antenatal support & information, health clubs with crèches, personal trainers, swimming pools, yoga)

Local leisure centres and maternity hospitals often hold exercise classes for new mothers

Guild of Postnatal Exercise Teachers
01453 884268
www.postnatalexercise.co.uk

Jo Charlton
020 8755 1460
Pilates-ante/post natal

Moves Fitness
01483 850057
Various locations in Surrey

Camberley
Pam Mates
01276 500232

Croydon
Liza Claxton
020 8654 6497

Dorking
Anne Clews
clews@chalkpit45.fsnet.co.uk

Guildford
Jo Yearwood
01483 232412

Teddington
Mums and Bumps
020 8943 0270

Sue Olsen
020 8367 6784

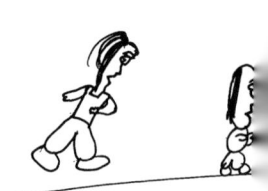

ex-pat advice

American Women's Club of London
68 Old Brompton Road, London, SW7
020 7589 8292

Focus Information Services
13 Prince of Wales Terrace, London, W8
020 7937 0050

eyes

Institute of Optometry
56-62 Newington Causeway, London, SE1
020 7234 9642

Liz May
020 8878 3686
Bates method

family planning

Brook
0800 0185 023
Pregnancy advice and contraception to under 25's

Contraceptive Education Helpline
Family Planning Association
020 7837 4044

Family Planning Asociation
Staines Health Centre, Knowle Green, Staines
01784 454135

Marie Stopes House
020 7388 0662

fancy dress

Toy shops often carry a range of outfits

mail order

Charlie Crow
01782 417133

Fairytales
PO Box 21220, London W9 1ZE. 020 7286 7142

Fancy Days
020 8675 9160

Hopscotch
61 Palace Road, London SW2 3LB
020 8674 9853
www.hopscotchmailorder.co.uk

Make Believe
020 8789 5194

Stompers
020 8942 3446
www.stompers.co.uk

retail

Ashtead
Abracadabra
51 The Street. 01372 273 829

Farnham
Measure for Measure
5 Cambridge Place, East Street. 01252 737332

Kingston-upon-Thames
Books Bits & Bobs
8 Richmond Road. 020 8546 6655

Leatherhead
Bookham Costume Galleries
Leatherhead Road, Great Bookham
01372 452 668
Thurs- Mon

Richmond
PICCOLO BELLA
6 Eton Street. 020 8948 8601
www.thetoy-station.com
Children's wear 0-6yrs. Dressing up clothes and accessories.

Teddington
MUM AND ME
61 High Street. 020 8255 0073
See advert under nearly new

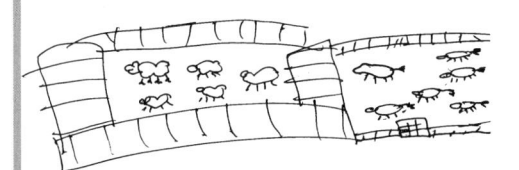

farms

(see also outings, parks & playgrounds, zoos)

Buckinghamshire
Odds Farm Park
Wooburn Common, High Wycombe
01628 520188
Jct 2, M40. Signposted from A4

Essex
Marsh Farm Country Park
South Woodham Ferrers. 01245 321552

Hertfordshire
Aldenham Country Park
Dagger Lane, Elstree. 020 8953 9602

Willows Farm Village
Coursers Road, London Colney, St Albans
01727 822106

farms are fun

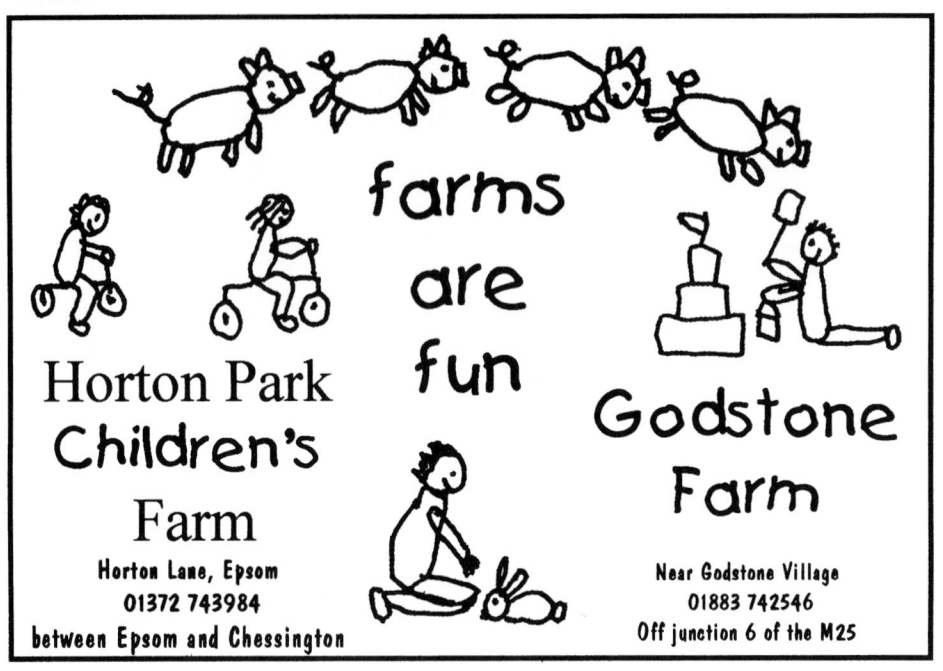

Horton Park Children's Farm
Horton Lane, Epsom
01372 743984
between Epsom and Chessington

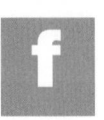

Godstone Farm
Near Godstone Village
01883 742546
Off junction 6 of the M25

farms (cont.)

Wimpole Hall Home Farm
Arrington, Royston. 01223 207257

Middlesex
Hounslow Urban Farm
Faggs Road, Feltham. 020 8751 0850
Spring/summer opening Feb 4th - Oct 31st
10am-4pm except Mondays (open bank holiday Mondays)

Surrey
Bocketts Farm Park
Young Street, Fetcham. 01372 363764

Deen City Farm
39 Windsor Avenue, Merton Abbey
020 8543 5300
9.30-5pm

GODSTONE FARM
Tilburstow Hill Road, Godstone
01883 742546
www.godstonefarm.co.uk

HORTON PARK CHILDREN'S FARM
Horton Lane, Epsom. 01372 743984
www.hortonpark.co.uk
See advert under outings

Losely Park Farm
Losely Farm Estate Offices. 01483 304440
Open Spring/Summer

fatherhood

(see also helplines)

Families Need Fathers
134 Curtain Road. 020 7613 5060

www.fathersdirect.com

Visit us at
www.babydirectory.com

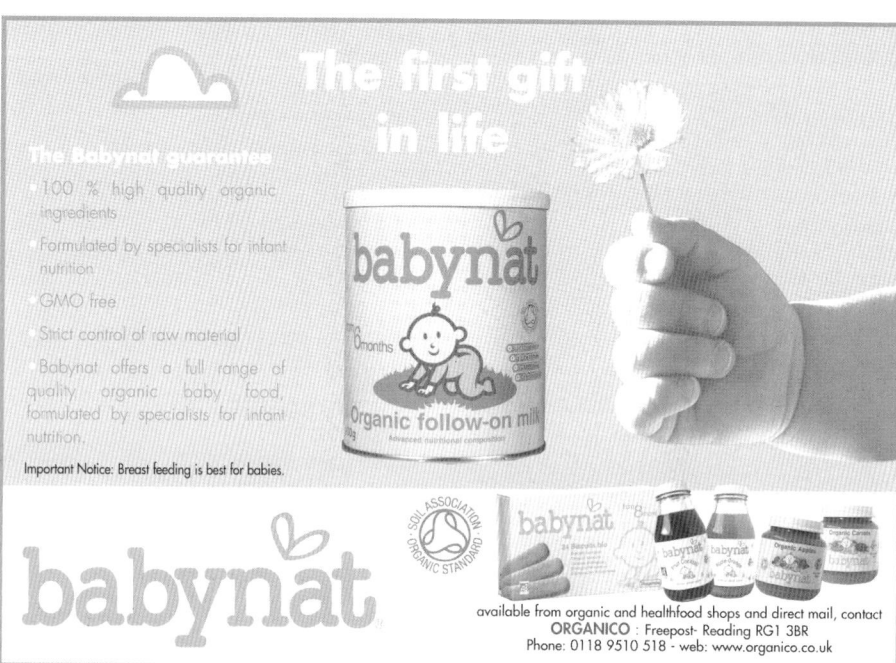

feng shui

Feng Shui Association
01273 693844
www.fengshuiassociation.co.uk

Twickenham
The Feng Shui Practice
11 Stafford Road. 020 8891 0794

financial advice

**TUNBRIDGE WELLS
EQUITABLE FRIENDLY SOCIETY**
Abbey Court, St John's Road,
Tunbridge Wells, Kent
01892 515353
www.twefs.co.uk

Chartwell Associates (UK) Ltd
80 High Street, Egham. 01784 434820

Family Assurance Friendly Society
0800 616695

Friends Provident
United Kingdom House, 72-122 Castle Street, Salisbury. 01722 318000

IFG Financial Services Ltd
Trinity House, Anderson Road, Swavesey, Cambridgeshire. 01954 233555

Invesco Europe
11 Devonshire Square, London. 020 7626 3434

John Charcol Ltd
0800 718191

Jump
0800 082 8180

Royston Fox
Russell Fox Nori, 117 Piccadilly, Mayfair, London. 020 7744 6556

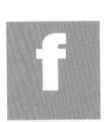

first aid courses

(see also safety advice)

Crêchendo Training
020 8772 8160
www.crechendo.co.
Will run courses for groups in your home

Twickenham
St John Ambulance Lifesaver
Clifton College. 020 8892 1026
Saturdays ½ day

flower remedies

Little Miracles
PO Box 3896, London, NW3 7DS
020 7431 6153

The Institute of Phytobiophysics
01534 738737
Call for list of therapists. Mail order available, including a birth harmony kit

food

(see also organics, pubs, restaurants)

BABYNAT
0118 951 0518
www.organico.co.uk
Organic follow-on milk availabe from organic & healthfood shops or direct mail
See advert on page 25

Truuuly Scrumptious Organic
Baby Food Ltd, Unit 2, Charmborough Farm, Charlton Road, Holcombe, Radstock
01761 239300
www.bathorganicbabyfood.co.uk
Frozen organic baby and toddler food, home deliveries

football

(see also leisure centres)

Football in the Community run weekend and holiday courses for 5yrs+

Kids Works
020 8755 1583
Age 3-10yrs. Sheen & Teddington

footprints

(see also ceramics)

FOOTPRINTS
baby-feet at home. 020 7736 2157
www.baby-feet.com
Create a lasting memento of your baby's footprints on pottery £29
See advert on page 13

french classes & clubs

LA JOLIE RONDE
01949 839715
info@lajolieronde.co.uk
www.lajolieronde.co.uk
French for children 3-11yrs. Classes throughout the UK

French & Spanish A La Carte
020 8946 4777

Le club français
020 408 3131
3-10yrs

Le Kinder Club
020 8943 5363
Richmond & Kingston. 3-9yrs

Hampton Hill
The Language Club
22 Cramer Road. 020 8288 1710
4-10yrs

Kew
Frère Jacques
020 7354 0589
3-11yrs

Richmond
La Petite Ecole
020 8948 6326

french language aids

1.2.3. Soleil
0845 085 0048
info@123-soleil.co.uk
www.123-soleil.co.uk
For a head start in French

german classes & clubs

Le Kinder Club
020 8943 5363
Richmond & Kingston. 3-9yrs

Croydon
German Saturday Schools
01959 571924

Richmond
German Saturday Schools
020 8942 5663

The German School
Douglas House, Petersham Road
020 8940 2510

gifted children

Gifted Monthly
28 Wallis Close, London. 0788 792 3165
info@giftedmonthly.com
www.giftedmonthly.com
Gifted child? Get your free issue of our newsletter today

National Association for Gifted Children
0870 770 3217

gifts

(see also mail order)

DODOPAD
PO Box 10507, London, N22 7WZ
0870 900 8004
www.dodopad.com
Indodispensible family organiser in desk, calendar & pocket formats - practical & fun - plus much more...

Glittergifts
sales@glittergifts.co.uk
www.glittergifts.co.uk
Unique, affordable, personalised, handmade gifts for every occasion. Beautifully packaged

GOLDEN HANDS, SILVER FEET LTD.
Unit G. Homesdale Centre,
216-218 Homesdale Road,
Bromley, Kent
www.goldenhands.co.uk

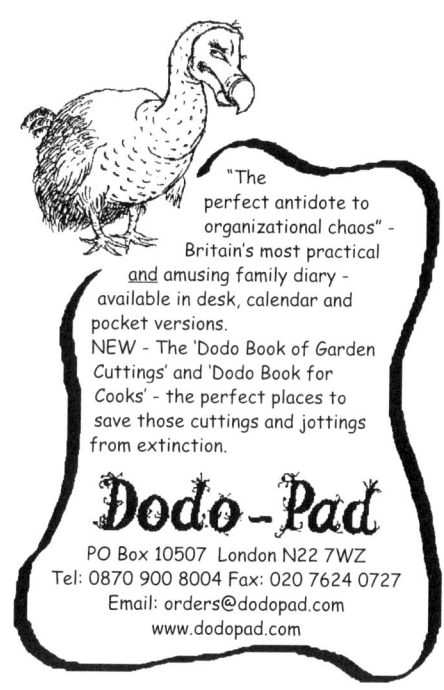

Happy Hands
7 Brockwell Park Row, Tulse Hill, London
020 8671 2020
info@happyhands.ws
www.happyhands.ws
Hand and foot prints and works of art preserved on ceramic tiles

I Love Balloons Ltd
020 8904 0004
www.Iloveballoons.co.uk
Beautiful balloons bouquet deliveries for newborn babies and birthdays

Little Angel
01473 323 146
www.littleangel.info
A beautiful keepsake box, contains a gift for mum, dad, baby and can include a gift for siblings. Starts at £45.00. Brands include Petit Bateau/Dior

---

"The perfect antidote to organizational chaos" - Britain's most practical <u>and</u> amusing family diary - available in desk, calendar and pocket versions.
NEW - The 'Dodo Book of Garden Cuttings' and 'Dodo Book for Cooks' - the perfect places to save those cuttings and jottings from extinction.

Dodo-Pad
PO Box 10507 London N22 7WZ
Tel: 0870 900 8004 Fax: 020 7624 0727
Email: orders@dodopad.com
www.dodopad.com

Please say you saw the ad in
The Local Baby Directory

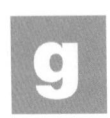

gifts (cont.)

Stork Express
PO Box 150, Amersham,
Buckinghamshire, HP7 0TH. 01494 434294
www.storkexpress.co.uk.
Baby gifts and baby gift baskets sent nationwide and worldwide

gym

(see also leisure centres)

Many local leisure centres offer gym classes

Kanga & Roo Club
020 8392 0125
3-5yrs. Craft & fitness classes

Camberley
TUMBLE TOTS
01276 62438
www.tumbletots.com
Call for locations in Camberley, Fleet, Mytchett and Farnham

Croydon
TUMBLE TOTS
020 8406 5200
karen@tumbletots.com/croydon
Call for location in Coulsdon, Sanderstead, Thornton Heath, Kenley, New Addington, Central Croydon and South Croydon

Dorking
TUMBLE TOTS
01372 273649
www.tumbletots.com
Call for location in Dorking, Leatherhead, Woking & Cobham

Ham
G&M Gym Club
020 8977 7251
4^1/$_2$ yrs+

Haslemere
TUMBLE TOTS
01483 420741
www.tumbletots.com
Call for locations in Godalming, Guildford, Shamley Green, Haslemere and Cranleigh

Oxted
TUMBLE TOTS
01892 655556
www.tumbletots.com
Call for locations in Oxted, E.Grinstead, Tunbridge Wells, Matfield, Rotherfield and Larkfield

Redhill
TUMBLE TOTS
01273 883782
www.tumbletots.com
Call for location in Horsham, Crawley, Redhill and Reigate

Richmond
Richmond Rompers
020 8878 8682

Sutton
TUMBLE TOTS
01737 352375
www.tumbletots.com
Call for locations in Epsom, Cheam, Banstead and Sutton

Teddington
G&M Gym Club
020 8977 7251
4^1/$_2$ yrs+

Twickenham
Kids Works
020 8755 1583
Gym clubs in Teddington, Sheen, Twickenham. 14mths-10yrs

TUMBLE TOTS
01932 568263
www.tumbletots.com
Call for location in Twickenham, Kingston-upon-Thames, Kew, Hampton & Chiswick

Weybridge
TUMBLE TOTS
01932 564512
www.tumbletots.com
Call for location in Weybridge, Walton on Thames, Esher, Addlestone, Sunbury, Shepperton, Byfleet, Hersham, West Moseley

Tumble Tots.
20 years of building self-confidence in Britain's children.

*T*umble Tots is the UK's leading national active play programme.

Since 1979, almost 1 Million children aged between six months & seven years have gained self-confidence and self-esteem at Tumble Tots through:

DEVELOPING PHYSICAL SKILLS OF AGILITY, BALANCE AND CO-ORDINATION.
DEVELOPING LANGUAGE WITH ACTION SONGS AND RHYMES.
HAVING FUN & MAKING FRIENDS IN A SAFE ENVIRONMENT.

Contacts & centres in your area:

Karen McGee
Tel: 020 8406 5200
Coulsdon, Caterham,
Norbury, Kenley,
Central Croydon,
South Croydon.

Nicky Spink
Tel: 01932 564 512
Addlestone, Walton on
Thames, Sunbury, West
Moseley, Thames Ditton,
Shepperton, Byfleet,
Weybridge, Hersham

Julie Eke
Tel: 01892 655556
Tunbridge Wells,
Oxted, Matfield,
Rotherfield,
Larkfield

Helen Jutting
Tel: 01932 568 263
Twickenham, Kew,
Kingston, Hampton,
Chiswick

Sue Knight
Tel: 01483 420 741
Godalming, Guildford,
Shamley Green,
Haslemere, Cranleigh

Gill Smith
Tel: 01372 273 649
Dorking,
Leatherhead, Woking,
Cobham

Lorraine Puttock
Tel: 01273 883 782
Redhill, Horsham,
Crawley, Reigate.

David Barker
Tel: 01276 62438
Camberley, Fleet,
Mychett

Nora Shipley
Tel: 01737 352 375
Cheam, Banstead,
Wallington, Epsom

For information on your nearest centre, contact:

0121 585 7003
www.tumbletots.com

hairdressers

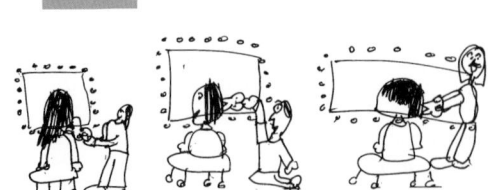

Many hairdressers have a special chair attachment, and offer a cheap cut for kids - though some can't be bothered so take your custom elsewhere!

health clubs with crèches

(see also exercise, leisure centres, swimming pools, personel trainers)

Local authority sports centres often provide crèches to supplement their sports activities

Brentford
Top Notch Health Club
Windsor Close. 020 8569 8225

Croydon
Cannons Health Club
020 8681 1885

Esporta Health & Rackets Club
Hannibal Way. 020 8681 1331

Ladies Own Health & Fitness
73 Northend. 020 8686 0111

Ewell
Dragons Health & Fitness Club
020 8393 6011

Farnham
Cannons Health Club
01252 747500

Kingston-upon-Thames
Holmes Place
Bentalls Centre. 020 8549 7700
Ozone cleaned swimming pool.
Crèche in Bentalls Centre

Esporta Health Club
Above Sainsburys. 020 8481 6000

LA Fitness
161 Clarence Street. 020 8943 0970

Mitcham
Cannons Leisure Centre
020 8640 8543

Richmond
Cannons Health Club
020 8948 3743

Cedars
144-150 Richmond Hill. 020 8332 1010

Ladies Own Health & Fitness
Kew Road. 020 8948 8411

Sunbury-on-Thames
HOLMES PLACE SUNBURY
The Avenue. 01932 755 750
kates@sunbury.hphc.co.uk
www.holmesplace.com
Children's memberships available, includes registered crèche, pool & ace activities

Surbiton
Cannons Health Club
020 8335 2999

Pinnacle
Simpson Way. 020 8335 2999

Sutton
Cannons Health Club
020 8770 7858

Ladies Own Health & Fitness
2a Mulgrave Road. 020 8661 1919

Teddington
Lensbury Club
Broom Road. 020 8614 6400
Closed to new family membership for 3 years

Thames Ditton
Colets Health & Fitness
St. Nicholas Road. 020 8398 7108

Twickenham
Cannons Health Club
020 8892 2251

West Byfleet
Cannons Health Club
01932 351835

Weybridge
St Georges Hill Health & Fitness
01932 843591

health food shops

(see also organic)

Banstead
Pumpkin Patch
10 High Street. 01737 371007

Brentford
Syon Park Farm Shop Ltd
Syon Park. 020 8847 2140

Camberley
Food For Thought
30-32 High Street. 01276 691996

Caterham-on-the-Hill
Village Health Foods
5b High Street. 01883 345633

Cheam
Healthfoods Cheam Village
60 The Broadway. 020 8643 5132

Cranleigh
Natural Life
Tudor House. 01483 272742

Croydon
Wholefood Shop
96 High Street. 020 8686 6167

Dorking
Aromantic
16 St Martins Walk. 01306 742005

East Horsley
Body & Soul Organic Foods
1 Parade Court. 01483 282868

Epsom
The Good Life
1 Waterloo Road. 01372 742095

Esher
Sloane Health Shop
50 High Street. 01372 465864

Guildford
Food For Thought
2/6 Haydon Place. 01483 533841

Haslemere
Haslemere Health Foods
71 Wey Hill

Hindhead
Grayshott Health Store
1 Headley Road. 01428 604046

Hounslow
Food for Thought
154 High Street. 020 8572 0310

Kew
Oliver's Wholefoods
5 Station Approach. 020 8948 3990

Kingston-upon-Thames
Food For Thought
7-8 Market Place. 020 8546 7806

Millenium Health Foods
29 The Bentalls Centre. 020 8549 8341

Oxted
Oxted Health Foods
75 Station Road East. 01883 730060

Purley
Purley Wholefoods
48 High Street. 020 8668 1293

Shepperton
Rawnsley Country Fresh Farm Shops
Squires Garden Centre. 01932 8761496

Surbiton
Pulses
372 Ewell Road. 020 8339 9069

Surbiton Whole Foods
14 Claremont Road. 020 8399 2772

Sutton
Good Life
207 High Street. 020 8770 1156

Twickenham
Healthy Harvest
Squires Garden Centre, Sixth Cross Road
020 8943 0692

Wallington
Noah Health Food Stores
4 South Parade. 020 8647 1724

Walton-on-Thames
Lifestyle Natural Health Centre
9 Hersham Centre. 01932 254624

helplines

If you can't find what you're looking for here, try the index at the back of the book

aids
Positively Women. 020 7713 0222

Sexual Health & National Health Helpline
0800 567123
Information on aids and sexually transmitted diseases

allergy
British Allergy Foundation. 020 8303 8583
www.allergyfoundation.com

anaphylaxis
Anaphylaxis Campaign. 01252 542029
www.anaphylaxis.org.uk
Severe allergic reactions, e.g. nuts

asthma
National Asthma Campaign. 020 7226 2260
www.asthma.org.uk

autism
National Autistic Society. 020 7833 2299
www.nas.org.uk

bedwetting
Bedwetting Education Advisory Line
0800 085 8189

Enuresis Resource & Information Centre (ERIC). 0117 960 3060
www.eric.org.uk

bereavement
Child Bereavement Trust. 01494 446648
www.childbereavement.org.uk

Child Death Helpline. 0800 282 986

CRUSE Bereavement Care. 020 8940 4818

Stillbirth and Neonatal Death Society (SANDS). 020 7436 7940
www.uk-sands.org
Information and support for bereaved parents

Visit us at
www.babydirectory.com

birth
Birth Crisis Network. 01865 300266

Birth Defects Foundation. 08700 707020

National Childbirth Trust. 0870 4448707

blindness
LOOK (National Federation of Families with Visually Impaired Children. 0121 428 5038

RNIB. 020 7391 2245

brain damage
British Institute for Brain Injured Children
01278 684060
www.bibic.org.uk

bullying
Anti-Bullying Campaign. 020 7378 1446
For children bullied at school

Kidscape. 020 7730 3300
www.kidscape.org.uk

caesarians
Caesarian Support Network. 01624 661269
6pm-10pm, weekends

cerebral palsy *See also main entry*
Cerebral Palsy Helpline (SCOPE)
0808 800 3333
www.scope.org.uk
Mon-Fri, 9am -9pm; w/e 2 -6pm

childcare
Daycare Trust. 020 7840 3350
National childcare campaign

Home-Start UK. 020 7388 6075
www.home-start.org

children
ChildLine. 0800 1111
www.childline.org.uk

cleft lip
Cleft Lip and Palate Association (CLAPA)
020 7431 0033
www.clapa.com

coeliac disease
Coeliac UK. 01494 437278

cot death
Cot Death Helpline. 0845 601 0234

h

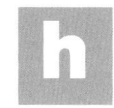

Cot Death Society. 01925 850086
www.cotdeathsociety.co.uk

Foundation for the Study of Infant Deaths
020 7233 2090
www.sids.org.uk/fsid

cruelty
NSPCC Child Protection Helpline
0800 800 500

crying babies
Serene (incorporating Cry-sis). 020 7404 5011
Helpline 8am-11pm

cystic fibrosis
Cystic Fibrosis Trust. 020 8464 7211
www.cftrust.org.uk

deafness
National Deaf Children's Society
020 7250 0123

diabetes
Diabetes UK
(ex-British Diabetes Association)
020 7323 1531
www.diabetes.org.uk

disability
Contact-A-Family. 020 7383 3555
www.cafamily.org.uk
Local parent support groups

Council for Disabled Children. 020 7843 6000
www.ncb.org.uk

Disability Alliance. 020 7247 8763
Advice on rights

Scope. 020 7619 7100
www.scope.org.uk/

divorce
Mediation in Divorce. 020 8891 6860

down's syndrome
Down's Heart Group. 01525 220379

Down's Syndrome Association. 020 8682 4001
www.dsa.uk.com

dyslexia
British Dyslexia Association. 0118 966 8251
See also reading difficulties

dyspraxia
Dyspraxia Foundation. 01462 454986
For help with 'Clumsy Child Syndrome'

eczema
National Eczema Society. 020 7388 4097
www.eczema.org

education
British Association for
Early Childhood Education. 020 7539 5400
www.early-education.org.uk

Children's Information Service. 0800 960296
www.childcarelink.gov.uk

Home Education Advisory Service
01707 371854
www.heas.co.uk

ISCis: London & South East. 020 7798 1560
www.iscis.uk.net/southeast

endometriosis
National Endometriosis Society
020 7222 2781
www.endo.org.uk

The SHE Trust
(Simply Holistic Endometriosis)
01522 519992
www.shetrust.org.uk

epilepsy
British Epilepsy Association. 0113 210 8800
www.epilepsy.org.uk

fatherhood
Families Need Fathers. 020 7613 5060
www.fnf.org.uk
Advice for non-custodial parents

formula milk
Baby Milk Action. 01223 464420
www.babymilkaction.org

fragile X
Fragile X Society. 01424 813147

health
Group B Strep Support. 01444 416176
www.gbss.org.uk

NHS Direct. 0845 4647
www.nhsdirect.nhs.uk
24-hr line

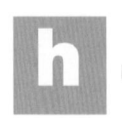

helplines (cont.)

Women's Health. 020 7251 6580
www.womenshealthlondon.org.uk
Gynaecological and sexual health. Reference library and advice

herpes
Herpes Viruses Association. 020 7609 9061

hyperactivity
Hyperactive Children's Support Group
01903 725182
10am-1pm

learning difficulties
British Institute for Learning Disabilities
01562 723010

marriage
National Family Mediation. 020 7383 5993

Relate: National Marriage Guidance
020 8367 7712
www.relate.org.uk

maternity
Assoc for Improvements in Maternity Services AIMS. 020 8390 9534
www.aims.org.uk

ME
Action for ME Pregnancy Network
01749 670799
www.afme.org.uk

meningitis
Meningitis Research. 08088 003344
www.meningitis.org

Meningitis Trust. 0845 600 0800
www.meningitis-trust.org.uk

miscarriage
Miscarriage Association. 01924 200799
www.miscarriageassociation.org.uk

motherhood
Meet a Mum Association (MAMA)
01761 433598
www.mama.org

multiple births
Multiple Births Foundation. 020 8383 3519
www.multiplebirths.org.uk

parenthood
National NEWPIN. 020 7358 5900

Parentline Plus. 0808 800 2222
www.parentlineplus.org.uk
For parents under stress

postnatal depression
Association for Postnatal Illness
020 7386 0868
www.apni.org

pre-eclampsia
Action on Pre-Eclampsia (APEX helpline)
020 8427 4217
Calls 10am-1pm

reading difficulties
National Advice Centre for Children with Reading Difficulties. 0845 604 0414

sexual abuse
SACCAA. 020 8950 7855

sick children
Action for Sick Children. 0800 074 4519

single parents
National Council for One-Parent Families
0800 185026
www.oneparentfamilies.org.uk

stammering
British Stammering Association
020 8983 1003
www.stammering.org

twins
Twins and Multiple Births. 01732 868 8000
Helpline only 7-11pm evenings and weekends. Weekdays: 0151 348 0020

violence
Women's Domestic Violence Helpline
0161 839 8574
www.wdvh.org.uk

working parents
Parents at Work. 020 7628 2128
www.parentsatwork.org.uk

hiring equipment

(see also nearly new shops, party equipment)

LITTLE STARS
33 Royston Park Road, Hatch End,
Pinner. 020 8621 4378/ 020 8537 0980
little.stars@virgin.net
www.littlestars.co.uk
Buy or hire your new baby equipment today

Chelsea Baby Hire
020 8946 9172

Nappy Express
020 8361 4040

West Horsley
Abacus Baby & Partyhire
01483 285142
Cots, highchairs, backpacks etc

holiday play schemes

Local councils often run grant-aided holiday schemes. Independent schools, leisure centres, swimming pools and private companies offer their own programmes. See also art, cookery, football, etc

Barracudas Multi-Activity Day Camps
Cobham, Croydon & Farnham. 5-14yrs

Campsters
020 755 1583
Multi-activity holiday camps. 3-10yrs
Teddington & Sheen.

Dorking
Adventure & Computer Holidays Ltd
P.O.Box 183. 01306 881299

East Molesey
Rosalita Edwards Montessori Nursery & Daycare
East Molesey Cricket Club. 020 8979 2542
5-8yrs

Horley
Cranbrook (C.A.T.S Club)
Coppingham Cottage, Balcome Road
01293 823163
4-16yrs

Old Woking
KIDSPORTS
Chris Lane Family Leisure Club, Westfield Avenue. 01483 722113
www.chrislane.com
Fun, unusual, activities for every holiday.
Ages 3 to 16yrs

Thames Ditton
Clubland Holiday Club
020 8224 1359

Tolworth
Playschemes
Knollmead Primary School. 020 8537 5208
3-6yrs

Worcester Park
Holiday Schemes
Green Lane School. 020 8337 6078

home birth

(see also antenatal support & information, midwives)

National Childbirth Trust branches often have a home birth support group. If you get no joy from your GP, contact your local hospital's Director of Midwifery *(see hospitals)* or an independent midwife *(see midwives)*

Home Birth Support Group
020 8525 0025

Home Birth Support Group (Twickenham NCT)
020 8255 1206
www.homebirth.org

AIMS (Association for Improvement in Maternity Service)
0870 765 1433
www.aims.org.uk

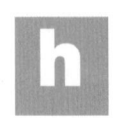

FARNHAM HOMEOPATHIC CHILDREN'S CLINIC
(01252) 713338

Digestive and sleep disturbances - Colic and teething difficulties
Recurrent coughs and colds - Pregnancy and labour difficulties

Claudia Demire BA L.C.H. RShom
Registered member of the Society of Homeopaths

homeopathy

(see also complementary health)

A gentle treatment that can be used on babies and pregnant women for a wide range of symptoms. Remedies are available at chemists and health shops, but if in doubt it is always best to consult a homeopath

A plethora of 'national' organisations representing homeopaths

College of Practical Homeopathy
020 8445 6123
For a list of medically qualified homeopaths, doctors and dentists

United Kingdom Homeopathic Medical Association
6 Livingstone Road, Gravesend, Kent
01474 560336

Helios Homeopathic Pharmacy
020 7379 7434
Do a great labour kit plus general first aid box

Ashford
Ashford Osteopathic Clinic
23 Feltham Road. 01784 255535

Camberley
Camberley Natural Therapy Centre
9 Tekels Park. 01276 23300
sue@kalicinska.freeserve.co.uk

Cheam
Brenda McBride
6 Albury Avenue. 020 8786 8812

Epsom
Robin Logan
Epsom Natural Health Clinic. 01372 729100

Farnham
CLAUDIA DEMIRE
Woodpeckers, 1 Beam Hollow
01252 713338
www.farnhamhomeopathicpractice.co.uk

Fulham
Jo Millican
020 7736 4086
Will do telephone consultations after the first visit

Hampton
Doy Dalling
020 8979 0497

Richmond
Richmond Pharmacy Clinic
82-86 Sheen Road. 020 8940 3930

Staines
T M Cook
Cygnet House. 01784 440467

Teddington
David Weiss
71 Cambridge Crescent. 020 8943 9573

Twickenham
Cathy Bland
Oak Lane Medical Centre. 020 8891 5762

Kay Gale
4 Baronsfield Road. 020 8286 4943

Sabine Grocholski/Roger Sharpley
020 8898 1952

The Maris Practice
13 Baylis Mews, Amyand Park Road
020 8891 3400
www.stellamaris.org

Walton-on-Thames
Rita McGovern
01932 248824

Please say you saw the ad in
The Local Baby Directory

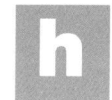

hospitals: dolls & teddies

The Doll and Teddy Hospital and Orphanage
Old Hill House, 53 Dover Street, Maidstone
01622 727020

The Doll's Hospital
17 George Street, Hastings. 01424 444117

Pinocchio
79 High Street, Teddington. 020 8977 8995
www.pinocchio-bearstore.com
Doll surgery

hospitals: NHS

In case of emergency call 999

Hospital for Sick Children
Great Ormond Street. 020 7405 9200
No accident & emergency. Specialist children's hospital

Action for Sick Children
1st floor, 300 Kingston Road, Wimbledon
0800 074 4519
Help for parents with children in hospital

Ashford
Ashford Hospital
London Road. 01784 884488
A&E

Camberley
Frimley Park Hospital
Portsmouth Road. 01276 604604
Maternity, A&E

Chertsey
St Peters Hospital
Guildford Road. 01932 872000
Maternity, A&E

Epsom
Epsom General Hospital
Dorking Road. 01372 735735
Maternity, A&E

Guildford
The Royal Surrey County Hospital
Egerton Road. 01483 571122
Maternity, A&E

Isleworth
West Middlesex University Hospital
Twickenham Road. 020 8560 2121
Maternity, A&E

Kingston-upon-Thames
Kingston Hospital
Galsworthy Road. 020 8546 7711
Maternity unit ext 2365
Maternity, A&E

Redhill
East Surrey Hospital
Canada Avenue. 01737 768511
Maternity, A&E

Teddington
Teddington Hospital
A & E (not 24 hrs)

hospitals: private maternity

Many of the NHS hospitals also have private wards, which may ensure some extra privacy and comfort. See above for contact details

London
The Portland Hospital for Women & Children
205-209 Great Portland Street, W1
020 7580 4400
www.theportlandhospital.com

BIRTH CENTRE
37 Coverton Road, Tooting, SW7
020 7498 2322
www.birthcentre.com
Give birth at home, in hospital or in our purpose-designed Birth Centre

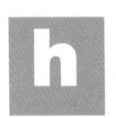

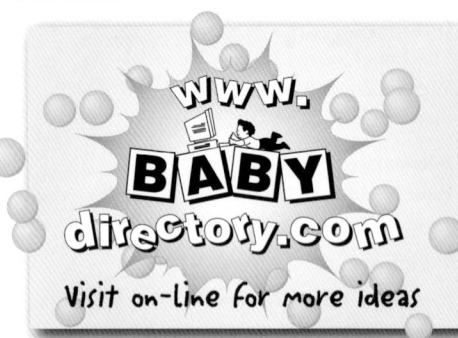

hotels & holidays

(see also ski companies, travel companies specialising in children, travel with kids)

The following offer special facilities for children and babies, ranging from crèches to child listening, playgrounds, pools, etc

Centerparcs Ltd
0990 200100

Avon
The Bath Spa Hotel
Sydney Road, Bath. 01225 444424

Channel Islands
Stocks Island Hotel
Manor Valley, Sark. 01481 832001

Clwyd
Oriel House Hotel
Upper Denbigh Road, St. Asaph. 01745 582716

Co.Durham
Redworth Hall Hotel
Redworth, Nr Newton Aycliffe. 01388 772442

Cornwall
FOWEY HOTEL
Hanson Drive, Fowey. 01726 833866
www.luxuryfamilyhotels.com
Play area, crèche, indoor pool

Bedruthan Steps Hotel
Mawgan Porth. 01637 860555

Carlyon Bay Hotel
Sea Road, St Austell. 01726 812304

Cawsand Bay Hotel
Cawsand, Torpoint. 01752 822425

Coombe Mill
St. Breward. 01208 850344

Long Cross Hotel
Trelights, Port Isaac. 01208 880243

Penmere Manor Hotel
Mongleath Road, Falmouth. 01326 211411

Polurrian
Mullion. 01326 240421

Sands Family Resort
Watergate Road, Porth. 01637 872864

Tredethy House Country Hotel
Helland Bridge, Bodmin. 01208 841262

Watergate Bay Hotel
Watergate Bay, Newquay. 01637 860543

Whipsiderry Hotel
Trevelgue Road, Porth, Newquay
01637 874777

Wringford Down Hotel
Cawsand. 01752 822287

Cumbria
Allerdale Court Hotel
Market Place, Cockermouth. 01900 823654

Armathwaite Hall Hotel
Nr. Keswick. 01768 776551

Castle Inn Hotel
Bassenthwaite, Keswick. 01768 776401

Hilton Keswick Lodore
Borrowdale Road, Keswick. 01768 777285

Devon
LANGSTONE CLIFF HOTEL
Mount Pleasant Road, Dawlish Warren, Dawlish. 01626 868000
reception@langstone-hotel.co.uk
www.langstone-hotel.co.uk
19 acres of woodland, children's suppers, indoor and outdoor pools, tennis, therapy rooms, go karts

THE KNOLL HOUSE
STUDLAND BAY

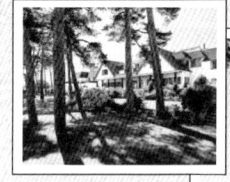

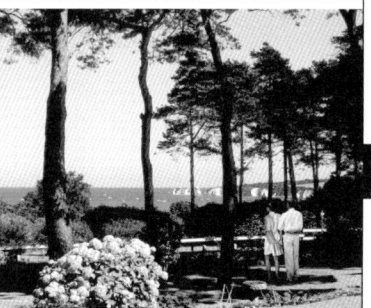

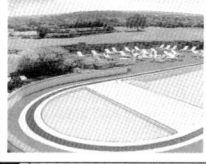

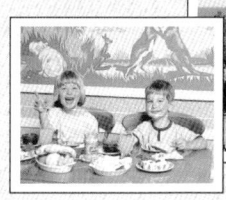

Established 1931

A peaceful oasis of traditional style
with a wonderful atmosphere for all ages

~

Easy access to three miles of golden beach
Outdoor pool (level deck), golf and tennis
Health Spa with plunge pool and sauna

~

Family suites of connecting rooms
Separate young children's restaurant
Playroom and fabulous safe Adventure Playground

~

Daily full board terms: £93 - £125
Children much less, by age
Excellent low season offers for young families:
£757 five nights full board, parents and two children

~

Open Easter - end October.   Dogs also very welcome

STUDLAND BAY
DORSET
BH19 3AX
TEL 01929 · 450450 FAX 01929 · 450423
Email: info@knollhouse.co.uk
Website: www.knollhouse.co.uk

ONLY 2 HOURS FROM HEATHROW

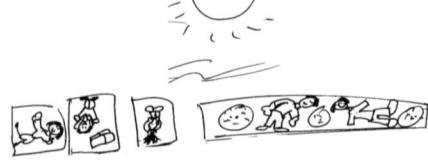

hotels & holidays (cont.)

Boswell Farm
Sidford. 01395 514162

The Bulstone Hotel
Higher Bulstone, Branscombe, Sidmouth
01297 680446

Radfords County Hotel
Dawlish. 01626 863322

Thurlestone Hotel
Thurlestone. 01548 560382

Dorset
KNOLL HOUSE
Studland Bay. 01929 450450
enquiries@knollhouse.co.uk
www.knollhouse.co.uk
Gardens, pools, tennis, golf, health spa, playroom, children's restaurant, adventure playground
See advert on page 39

MOONFLEET MANOR
Moonfleet, Nr Weymouth. 01305 786948
www.luxuryfamilyhotels.com
Play area, crèche, extensive leisure facilities including indoor pool

Chine Hotel
25 Boscombe Spa Road, Bournemouth
01202 396234

Fairfields Hotel
Studland Bay. 01929 450224

Hotel Buena Vista
Pound Street, Lyme Regis. 01297 442494

Sandbanks Hotel
15 Banks Road, Sandbanks, Poole
01202 707377

Dyfed
Hotel Penrallt
Aberporth, Cardigan. 01239 810227

East Lothian
Maitlandfield House Hotel
24 Sidegate, Haddington. 01620 826513

Essex
Churchgate Manor Hotel
Churchgate Street, Old Harlow. 01279 420246

Flintshire
St. David's Park Hotel
Ewloe. 01244 520800

Gloucestershire
Calcot Manor
Tetbury. 01666 890391

Gwynedd
Trefeddian Hotel
Aberdyfy. 01654 767213

Hampshire
Watersplash Hotel
The Rise, Brockenhurst. 01590 622344

Hertfordshire
Marriott Hanbury Manor
Nr Sandridge, Ware. 01920 487722

Inverness
Polmaily House Hotel
Drumnadrochit, Loch Ness. 01456 450343

Isle of Wight
The Clarendon Hotel - The Wight Mouse Inn
Chale. 01983 730431

Priory Bay Hotel
Eddington Road, St. Helens
01983 613146

Isles of Scilly
St Martin's on the Isle
Lower Town, St Martin's. 01720 422092

Kent
The Hythe Imperial
Hythe. 01303 267441

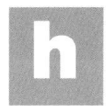

Kinross-shire
The Green Hotel
2 The Muirs, Kinross. 01577 863467

Lancashire
St. Ives Hotel
St. Anne's on Sea. 01253 720011

Leicestershire
Field Head Hotel
Markfield Lane, Markfield. 01530 245454

London
Charoscuro at Townhouse
24 Coptic Street, WC1. 020 7636 2731

Days Inn Hotel
54 Kennington Road, SE1. 020 7922 1331

London County Hall Travel Inn Capital
Belvedere Road, SE1. 0870 238 3300

myhotel
11-13 Bayley Street, Bedford Square, WC1
020 7667 6040

Norfolk
Heath Farm House B & B
Homersfield, Harleston. 01986 788417

North Devon
Saunton Sands Hotel
Nr Braunton. 01271 890212

Northumberland
Granary Hotel
Links Road, Amble. 01665 710872

Ryecroft Hotel
Ryecroft Way, Wooler. 01668 281459

Perthshire
Gleneagles Hotel
Auchterarder. 0800 328 4010
Playground, crèche

Stronvar House Scottish Vacations
Balquhidder. 01877 384688

Shropshire
Redfern Hotel
Cleobury Mortimer. 01299 270395

South Devon
Gara Rock
East Portlemouth, nr Salcombe. 01548 842342

Suffolk
ICKWORTH HOTEL
Nr Bury St Edmonds. 01284 735350
www.luxuryfamilyhotels.com
East wing of Ickworth House, within 1,800 acre National Trust estate. Indoor pool and crèche

Sussex
Family-Friendly Bed & Breakfast
Coombe Barn, Lewes. 01273 477388

Warwickshire
Lea Marston Hotel
Haunch Lane, Lea Marston. 01675 470468

Wiltshire
WOOLLEY GRANGE HOTEL
Woolley Green, Bradford on Avon
01225 864705
www.luxuryfamilyhotels.com
Play area, crèche, outdoor pool, bicycles

Old Bell
Abbey Row, Malmesbury. 01666 822344

Worcestershire
Evesham Hotel
Coopers Lane, Off Waterside, Evesham
01386 765566

Worcs
Holdfast Cottage Hotel
Welland, Nr Malvern. 01684 310288

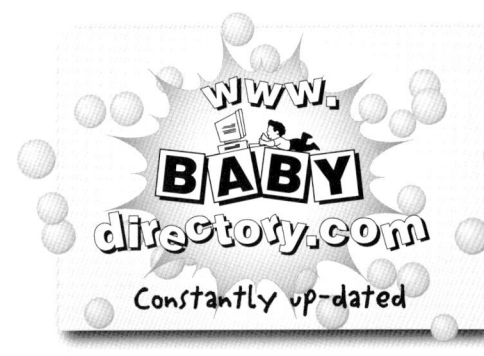

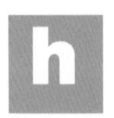

Transform your experience of pregnancy and childbirth with self hypnosis.

Benefit from relaxation and feel in control. Enjoy natural, drug-free pain relief and easier labour. Conquer morning sickness or 'baby blues'. Learn the simple and safe techniques of self hypnosis, without being hypnotised, on a short course specifically designed for mums-to-be.

Call Phillipa Nowell clinical hypnotherapist on 020-8572-0784

hypnotherapy

Can be useful for relaxation techniques during labour. Also used in smoking cessation and in the treatment of phobias. Self-hypnosis cassettes are available in some health shops and from practioners.

British Hypnotherapy Association
67 Upper Berkeley Street, London
020 7723 4443

Epsom
J.Edward Smith
9a Roseberry Road. 01372 278597

Esher
Susan Ratcliffe
Woodside House, Station Approach
020 8398 4333

Guildford
Robin Lee
Garden Croft Beech Lawn. 01483 455764

Hounslow
PHILIPPA NOWELL
44 Dene Avenue. 020 8572 0784
Member of the British Society of Clinical Hypnosis

London
Pauline Grant
020 8555 3698
Hypnobirtherapy

New Malden
Acorn Therapy Centre
7 Greenlaw Gardens. 020 8949 4573
Smoking cessation

Sutton
Michael Cohen
12 Fairfield Court. 020 8643 4925
Workshops and cassettes available

Thornton Heath
Dr C.O Murray
3 Lucerne Road. 020 8683 2649

Virginia Water
Molly Balaban
Glenwood House. 01784 431432

Wallington
Colin Flaherty
61 Stafford Road. 020 8669 5555

West Byfleet
J.L Golding
1 Blackwood Close. 01932 341055

Please say you saw the ad in **The Local Baby Directory**

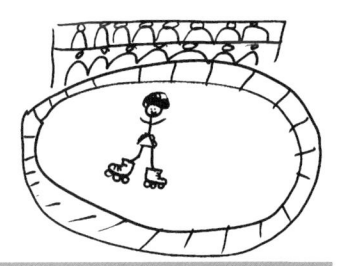

ice rinks

Guildford
Guildford Spectrum Leisure Complex
Guildford Spectrum, Parkway. 01483 443322

Streatham
Streatham Ice Arena
386 Streatham High Road. 020 8769 7771

indoor adventure playcentres

Local leisure centres may also have indoor play areas

Brentford
Little Tikes
Brentford Fountain Leisure Centre, Chiswick High Road. 020 8994 9596

Snakes & Ladders
Syon Park, London Road. 020 8847 0946
Parties and events

Camberley
Kids For Life
Bassett House, 5 Southwell Park Road
01276 684508

East Molesey
Bouncy Tots
Old Tiffonians Sports Centre, Summer Avenue
020 8398 1444
10-5pm, Mon-Fri

Epsom
Rainbow Circus
The Rainbow Centre, East Street. 01372 748725
Under 5's area plus circus area

Feltham
Jungle Jim's
Leisure West, Browells Lane. 020 8867 0500

Guildford
Rokers Little Angels
Fairlands Farm, Aldershot Road. 01483 236667
2-11yrs, max. ht. 1.5m

Horley
Air Balloon
60 Brighton Road. 01293 823726

Hounslow
Heathrow Gymnastic Club
Green Lane. 020 8569 5069
9-1pm Sat, 10-4pm Mon –Thurs, 3-8yrs

Richmond
Lollipop Club
Old Deer Park. 020 8332 7436
Term time only. 0-5yrs

Woking
Funky Forest
Hermitage Road. 01483 474312

Swingtime Indoor Adventure Play
Goldwater Lodge, Goldsworth Park,
Wishbone Way. 01483 799700

infertility

Assisted Conception
The Woking Nuffield Hospital, Shores Road, Woking. 01483 227800

CHILD - National Infertility Support Network
01424 732361

Concept Group
26 Church Street, Hampton. 020 8941 6652
Also hire Tens machines and run bereavement groups

Foresight
28 The Paddock, Godalming. 01483 427839

Human Fertilisation and Embryology Authority
Paxton House, 30 Artillery Lane, London E1
020 7377 5077

Don't forget to visit www.babydirectory.com

internet
(see also web sites)

Try your local library – the wealthier ones may offer terminals, with easy buggy access. Don't forget to look us up on
www.babydirectory.com

italian
(see also french clubs & classes)

Italian Day Nursery
174 Clapham Road, Clapham. 020 7735 3058

learning difficulties
(see also helplines)

Willoughby Hall Dyslexia Centre
1 Willoughby Road, London, NW3
020 7794 3538
6-12yrs

David Mulhall Centre
31 Webbs Road, London, SW11
020 7223 4321

left-handedness

Anything Lefthanded
020 8770 3722

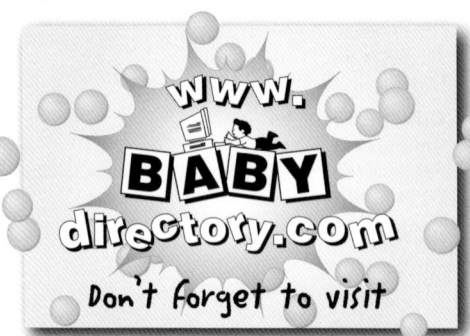

legal advice

Your local Citizen's Advice Bureau is a good starting point. The local library reference department may also be able to help

Children's Legal Centre
01206 873820

Education Law Association
01303 211570
For a list of solicitors in your area

leisure centres
(see also health clubs with crèches, swimming pools)

Addlestone
Abbeylands Sports Centre
School Lane. 01932 858966

Camberley
Arena Leisure Centre
Grand Avenue. 01276 28787
Swimming pool and crèche

Tomlinscote Sports Centre
Tomlinscote Way, Frimley. 01276 670316

Carshalton
Westcroft leisure Centre
Westcroft Road. 020 8770 4800
Swimming pool & soft play area

Caterham
de Stafford Sports Centre
Burntwood Lane. 01785 257081

Chessington
Chessington Sports & Leisure Centre
Garrison Lane. 020 8974 2277

Cranleigh
Cranleigh Leisure Centre
Village Way, High Street. 01483 274400
Crèche

Dorking
Dorking Swimming centre
Reigate Road. 01306 876661

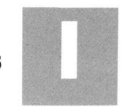

Egham
Egham Sports Centre
Vicarage Road. 01784 437695
Childrens soft play area

Epsom
Rainbow Leisure Centre
East Street. 01372 749606

Farnham
Farnham Sports Centre
East Street. 01252 723208
Swimming pool, crèche

Godalming
Godalming Leisure Centre
Broadwater Park, Summers Road
01483 417282

Guildford
Guildford Spectrum Leisure Complex
Guildford Spectrum, Parkway. 01483 443322

Horley
Oakwood Sports Centre
Balcombe Road. 01293 822238
After school clubs and half term activities

Kingston-upon-Thames
The Kingfisher Leisure Centre
Fairfield Road. 020 8546 1042
Ante/post natal classes, parent & baby sessions

Leatherhead
Leatherhead Leisure Centre
Guildford Road. 01372 377674

Mitcham
Canons Leisure Centre
Madeira Road. 020 8640 8543

Lavender Park & College Pavillion
Lavender Avenue. 020 8646 7362

New Malden
Malden Centre
Blagden Road. 020 8547 6601
Yoga, crèche, tots fun time

North Cheam
Cheam Leisure Centre
Malden Road. 020 8770 4830
Swimming pool, pool parties

Richmond
Springhealth Leisure Club
Pools on the Park, Old Deer Park, Twickenham Road. 020 8940 0561

South Croydon
Monks Hill Sports Centre
Farnborough Avenue. 020 8651 0984

Staines
Spelthorne Leisure Centre
Knowle Green. 01784 493493

Sunbury-on-Thames
Sunbury Leisure Centre
Nursery Road. 01932 772287

Surbiton
Tolworth Recreation Centre
Fullers Way N., North Tolworth. 020 8391 0684

Tadworth
Courtney's at Banstead Sports Centre
Merland Rise. 01737 361933
Swimming pool

Teddington
Teddington Sports Centre
Broom Road. 020 8977 0598
Toddler gym times

Walton-on-Thames
Elmbridge Leisure Centre
Waterside Drive. 01932 243863

Whitton
Whitton Sports Centre
Percy Road. 020 8898 7795
Toddler gym times

Woking
Woking Leisure Centre
Kingsfield Road. 01483 771122
Swimming pool and soft play area

Please say you saw the ad in
The Local Baby Directory

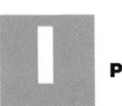

libraries

(see also toy libraries)

You and your children can join local libraries free of charge on proof of residence and borrow books, videos and cassettes. A fantastic resource, libraries are also a good source of local information. Days and times refer to under 5 storytime sessions. Some libraries run additional activity classes in the school holidays

Addlestone Library
Church Road. 01932 843648

Ashford Library
Church Road. 01784 253651
1st & 3rd Thurs of the month, 2pm

Ashtead Library
Woodfield Road. 01372 275875

Bagshot Library
High Street. 01276 473759

Banstead Library
The Horshoe, Bolters Lane. 01737 351271

Bedfont Library
639 Staines Road. 020 8890 6173
Thurs 2.15pm

Bookham Library
Townshott Close. 01372 454440

Bramley Library
High Street. 01483 892510

Brentford Library
Boston Manor Road. 020 8560 8801
Thurs 2.30pm

Byfleet Library
High Road. 01932 345274

Camberley Library
Knoll Road. 01276 63184

Carshalton Library
The Square. 020 8647 1151

Caterham Valley Library
Stafford Road. 01883 343580

Chertsey Library
Guildford Street. 01932 564101

Cobham Branch Library
Cedar Road. 01932 863292

Coulsdon Library
Brighton Road. 020 8660 1548

Cranford Library
Bath Road. 020 8759 0641
Mon 2.30pm

Cranleigh Library
High Street. 01483 272413

Dorking Library
Pippbrook. 01306 882948

Egham Library
High Street. 01784 433904

Epsom Library
17 The Parade. 01372 721707

Esher Library
Old Church Path. 01372 465036

Ewell Court Library
Lakehurst Road, Ewell. 020 8393 1069

Ewell Library
Bourne Hall, Spring Street. 020 8394 0951

Farnham Library
28 West Street. 01252 716021

Feltham Library
210 The Centre, High Street. 020 8890 3506
Tues 2.30pm

Frimley Green Library
Beech Road, Frimley Green. 01252 835530

Godalming Library
Bridge Street. 01483 422743

Grayshott Library
Village Hall, Headley Road. 01428 606256

Guildford Library
77 North Street. 01483 568496

Ham Library
Ham Street. 020 8940 8703
Thurs 2.30pm

Visit us at
www.babydirectory.com

Hampton Library
Rosehill. 020 8979 5110
Tues 2.15pm

Hampton Hill Library
Windmill Road. 020 8979 3705
Wed 2.15pm

Hampton Wick Library
Bennet Close. 020 8977 1559
Wed 3.45pm

Haslemere Library
91 Weyhill. 01428 642907

Heathfield Branch Library
Percy Road, Whitton. 020 8894 1017
Sat 10.30am

Hersham Library
Molesey Road. 01932 226968

Hook & Chessington Library
Hook Road, Chessington. 020 8397 4391

Horley Library
Victoria Road. 01293 784141

Horsley Library
Parade Court, Ockham Road South, East Horsley. 01483 283870

Hounslow Library
Treaty Centre. 020 8583 4545
Tues 2.15-3.00pm

Isleworth Library
Twickenham Road. 020 8560 2934
Mon 2.30pm

Kew Library
106 North Road. 020 8876 8654
Fri 2.30pm

Kingston Library
Fairfield Road. 020 8547 6400
Mon 2.15pm, Thurs 10.30am

Kingston School's Library Service
King Charles Centre, Hollyfield. 020 8390 5164

Knaphill Library
High Street. 01483 473394

Leatherhead Library
The Mansion, Church Street. 01372 373149

Lightwater Library
83a Guildford Road. 01276 452587

Lingfield Library
The Guest House, Vicarage Lane. 01342 832058

Merstham Library
Weldon Way. 01737 642471

Middleton Circle Library
Green Wrythe Lane. 020 8648 6608

Mitcham Library
London Road. 020 8648 4070
Mon 2.15-2.45pm

Morden Library
Merton Civic Centre, London Road
020 8545 4040
Fri 2.15-2.45pm

New Addington Library
Central Parade. 01689 841248

New Malden Library
Kingston Road. 020 8547 6540

Osterley Library
St Marys Crescent. 020 8560 4295
Mon 2.30pm

Oxted Library
12 Gresham Road. 01883 714225

Pollards Hill Library
South Lodge Ave. 020 8764 5877
Thurs 10.45-11.15am

Purley Library
Banstead Road. 020 8660 1171

Redhill Library
18-20 London Road. 01737 763332

Reigate Library
Bancroft House, Bancroft Road. 01737 244272

Richmond Library
The Little Green. 020 8940 0981
Thurs 2.15pm

Shepperton Library
High Street. 01932 225047

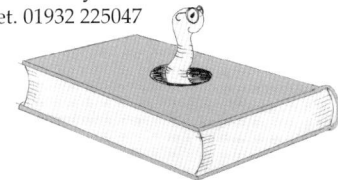

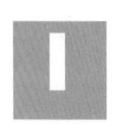

libraries (cont.)

Staines Library
Friends Walk. 01784 454430

Sunbury Library
The Parade, Staines Road West. 01932 225047

Surbiton Library
Ewell Road. 020 8399 2331
Mon 2.15-2.45pm

Sutton Central Library
St Nicholas Way. 020 8770 4700

Teddington Library
Waldegrave Road, Teddington. 020 8997 1284
Fri 2.15pm. Tiny Teddies storytime (18mths-3yrs) 1st Tues of the month 11am

Thornton Heath Library
Bridgestock Road. 020 8684 4432

Tolworth Community Library
37-39 The Broadway. 020 8339 6950
Tues 2.15pm

Twickenham District Library
Garfield Road. 020 8892 8091
Tues 2.15pm

Virginia Water Library
Station Parade. 01344 843388

Wallington Library
Shotfield. 020 8770 4900

Walton-on-Thames Library
High Street. 01932 224818

Warlingham Library
Shelton Avenue. 01883 6222479

West Barnes Library
Station Road. 020 8942 2635
Mon 2.15-2.45pm

West Byfleet Library
The Corner. 01932 343955

West Molesey Library
The Forum, Walton Road. 020 8979 6348

Weybridge Library
Church Street. 01932 843812

Whitton Library
Nelson Road. 020 8894 9828
Tues 2.15pm

Woking Library
Gloucester Walk. 01483 770591

Worcester Park Library
Windsor Road. 020 8337 1609

Wraysbury Library
The Green. 01784 482431

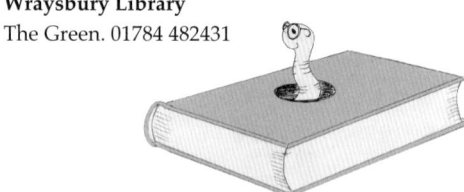

lice

NATURAL SCIENCE.COM LTD
Lindslade House, Middleton Street,
Llandrindod Wells, Powys
01597 823964
lucyabear@btconnect.com
www.lice.co.uk
Nice'n Clear Head Lice lotion - safe, effective, 10 minutes per application

linens

(see also sleeping bags)

COTTON FLEECE BLANKETS
Hippychick Ltd, Barford Gables, Spaxton, Somerset. 01278 671461
sales@hippychickltd.co.uk
www.hippychickltd.co.uk
100% natural cotton fleece baby blankets in a wonderful array of colours

babybabycompany
020 8876 3153

Visit us at www.babydirectory.com

www.babydirectory.com   The Local Baby Directory - *Surrey & S. Middlesex*   **Page 49**

Subscribe to your local Families Magazine

London area:
Families South West
Families South East
Families North
Families North West
Families West
Families Upon Thames
Families East
Elsewhere:
Thames Valley
Families Edinburgh
Families Liverpool

Ask for a free sample.

Families newsletters are packed full of local info: (new shops, new services, new playgroups, etc), features (parties, nurseries, etc) plus a fantastic Out & About listing.

Written by mothers who have lived in the area for years.

editor@FamiliesMagazine.co.uk
for information or to ask about
franchise opportunities.
020 8696 9680

Send £15.50 payable to Families, PO Box 4302, SW16 1ZS, stating which edition you require.
Also available free in after-school clubs, nurseries and elsewhere.

Online parenting: **www.FamiliesMagazine.co.uk** over a million hits a month!

The Great Little Trading Co.
Practical products for parents and kids

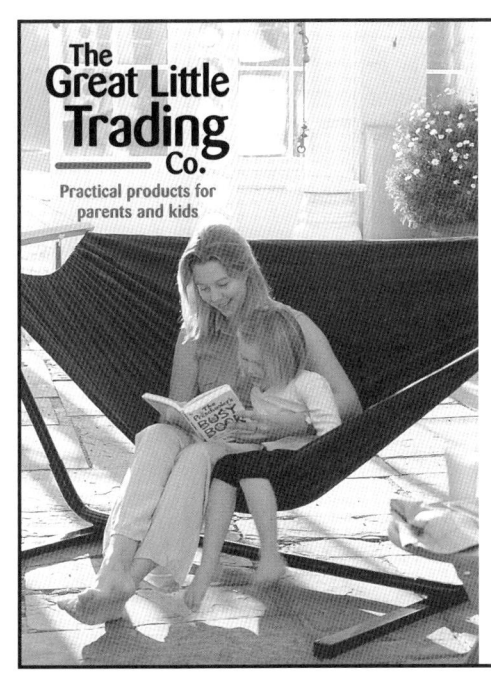

The Great Little Trading Company has hundreds of innovative and practical products to make your life as a parent easier. Our high quality products include:

- travel & holiday essentials
- childrens' furniture & storage ideas
- kitchen & bathroom accessories
- indispensable health & safety items
- imaginative play & gift ideas
  & much, much more.

For a FREE catalogue call
08702 41 40 81
www.gltc.co.uk

GLBD1

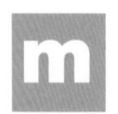

magazines

Families upon Thames
PO Box 425, KT12 5AG. 01932 883304

Hullaballoo
PO Box 32228, W5 1HY. 020 8991 0008

Parents' Directory
01243 527605

Parents' Guide
Studio 234, Bon Marché Centre,
241-251 Ferndale Road, SW9 8BJ. 020 7733 4955

mail order

mail order: accessories

GOO-GOO
07002 466 466
direct@goo-goo.com
www.goo-goo.com
Functional children's accessories,
see shoes, clothing, mail order: clothing

BONNE NUIT
020 8871 1472
sales@bonne-nuit.co.uk
www.bonne-nuit.co.uk
Beautiful French baby sleeping bags available in 3 sizes (0-4 years). Winter & summer collection. Call for brochure or stockist, or order online

www.pottypaper.com
Potty training starter kit

mail order: baby goods

GREAT LITTLE TRADING COMPANY
124 Walcot Street, Bath. 0870 2414081
cat@gltc.co.uk
www.gltc.co.uk
Hundreds of practical products designed to make your life as a parent a little bit easier

WWW.SMILECHILD.CO.UK
PO Box 274, Cheltenham,
Gloucester GL53 7YP. 0800 1956 982
info@smilechild.co.uk
www.smilechild.co.uk
Funky fashion, wooden toys, natural cosmetics, organics, eco-nappies and more

Mothercare Direct
01923 240365

The Nursery Emporium plc
Grower Court, New Road, Bromham,
Chippenham, Wiltshire. 01380 859171

mail order: clothing

GOO-GOO
07002 466 466
direct@goo-goo.com
www.goo-goo.com
Cocoon - new-born superfine and supersoft merino wool garments. Machine washable of course!

JOJO MAMAN BEBE
0870 241 0560
www.jojomamanbebe.co.uk
Great maternity wear, adorable baby & children's clothes, nursery products & toys - we're all you need

Silkstory
3 National Terrace, Bermondsey Wall East,
London. 0800 150874

mail order: gifts

LITTLE ANGEL
01473 323146
www.littleangel.info
A beautiful keepsake box, contains a gift for mum, dad, baby and can include a gift for siblings. Starts at £45.00. Brands include Petit Bateau/Dior

mail order: nursery furniture

DRAGONS OF WALTON STREET
020 7589 3795
Hand-painted children's furniture

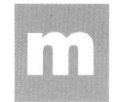

Little Stars
020 8621 4378/020 8537 0980
www.littlestars.co.uk
Buy or hire your new baby equipment today

HOUSE OF WINKLE
Offa House, Offa Street, Hereford
01432 268018
www.willeywinkle.co.uk
Organic mattresses and bedding

mail order: shoes

BOBUX
07002 466466
www.goo-goo.com
direct@goo-goo.com
Original soft leather shoes for under twos with stayonability!

SHOO SHOOS
Hippychick Ltd, Barford Gables, Spaxton, Somerset. 01278 671461
sales@hippychickltd.co.uk
www.hippychickltd.co.uk
Imaginative and refreshingly different, soft leather baby shoes (0-24 months)

SOLE MANIA
07002 466466
www.goo-goo.com
direct@goo-goo.com
Durable washable leather slippers for unstoppable nippers aged 2ish to 90ish!

STARCHILD SHOES
109 Paget Street, Loughborough, Leics
01509 550714
janet@star-child.co.uk
www.star-child.co.uk
Soft leather babies' shoes that really do stay on...

mail order: toys

Insect Lore Europe
PO Box 1420, Kiln Farm, Bucks. 01908 563338
Butterfly kits and other equipment

Mulberry Bush Ltd
Freepost SEA 4193, Billingshurst, West Sussex
01403 754400

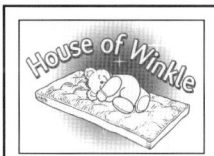

Maufacturers of the famous Willey Winkle products
Mattresses and Bedding in Organic and Luxury Wool for Adults and Children
The Willey Winkle Collection for moses baskets, cribs and cots all finished in 100% cotton ticking.
Scientifically Tested Mattress Materials
01432 268018
www.willeywinkle.co.uk
Designed & Crafted by Jeff Wilkes since 1969
Supporters of The Campaign Against Cot Death

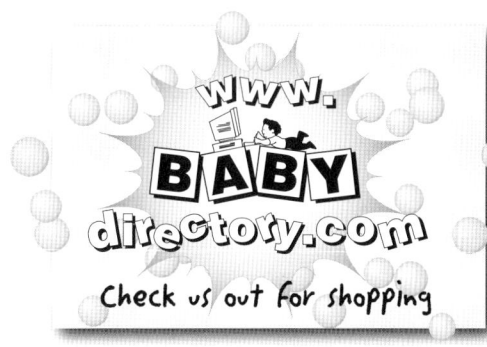

manufacturers & suppliers

Baby Dan UK
Nilebank Offices, 10 Beach Priory Gardens, Birkdale, Southport, Lancashire. 01704 502575

BabyBjorn AB
31-33 Park Royal Road. 0870 1200 543

Bambino Mio Ltd
12 Stavely Way, Brixworth, Northampton
01604 883777

Bebe Confort
Dyehouse Lane, Brighouse, West Yorkshire
01484 401802

Bebecar (UK) Ltd.
Bebecar House, Mill Hill Industrial Estate, Flower Lane, Mill Hill. 020 8201 0505

Brevi (Trend Europa Ltd.)
Unit D3, Rosehill Industrial Estate, Tern Hill, Shropshire. 01630 638978

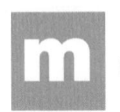

manufacturers & suppliers (cont.)

Brio Wonderland Ltd.
4 Nicholas Court, Nicholas Street Mews, Chester. 01706 750853

Cheeky Rascals
The Briars, Petworth Road, Witley, Surrey 01428 682489

Chicco UK Ltd.
Prospect Close, Kirkby-in-Ashfield, Notts 01623 750870

Cosatto (sales) Ltd.
Wollaston Way, Burnt Mills, Basildon, Essex 01268 722800

Fisher Price Nursery Products
Maclaren Limited, Station Works, Long Buckby, Northampton. 01327 842662

Galt Toys Ltd.
Brookfield Road, Cheadle, Cheshire 0161 428 9111

Graco Children's Products Ltd.
1 Hoverfields Avenue, Burnt Mills Industrial Estate, Basildon, Essex. 0870 909 0510

Jackel International Ltd.
Dudley Lane, Cramlington, Northumberland 0191 250 1864

Mamas & Papas Ltd.
Colne Bridge Road, Huddersfield, West Yorkshire. 01484 438200

Maxi-Cosi UK
Isopad House, Shenley Road, Borehamwood, Herts. 020 8236 0707

Silver Cross Ltd.
Otley Road, Guiseley, Leeds. 01943 876177

Stokke UK Ltd.
154 High Street, West Drayton, Middlesex 01753 655873

Tomy UK Ltd.
Wells House, 231 High Street, Sutton, Surrey 020 8661 4400

martial arts

Epsom
Martial Arts Centre
Alexandra Park. 07771 627292
3yrs+

Twickenham
Busen
9 King Street. 020 8892 3338

massage for baby & mother

(see also complementary health)

BABY BLISS
020 8568 4913

MARGUERITE & DECLAN BOWERS-CLARK
020 8336 1532
'From Bumps to Babies'. Also runs baby massage workshops in S.W.London

MILLPOND
020 8444 0040
www.mill-pond.co.uk
Discover the joys of baby massage, gentle solutions to colic, sleeplessness, etc

TOUCHING LIVES
10 Uxbridge Road, Hampton
020 8979 6261
touchinglives@ukgateway.net
www.touchinglives.co.uk
A holistic practitioner, working very much with balancing the natural energy within the body, concentrating on relieving stress in order to promote good health in both baby and adults alike

BodyCalm Therapeutic Massage for Women
01483 765300
Treatment in your own home. Also runs workshops

Camberley Natural Therapy Centre
9 Tekels Park. 01276 23300
sue@kalicinska.freeserve.co.uk

Crêchendo Training
020 8772 8160
www.crechendo.co.
Will run courses for groups in your home

Caroline Goodenough-Jones
01932 711930

Susan Grinnall
020 8395 2090

Claire Hunting
01372 274566

Janine Healey
01737 550190
Also runs baby massage workshops

Sara Kettle
020 8669 0205

Hilary Lewin
01306 730793

Anna Moore
Neal's Yard Remedies,
15 King Street, Richmond
020 8948 9248

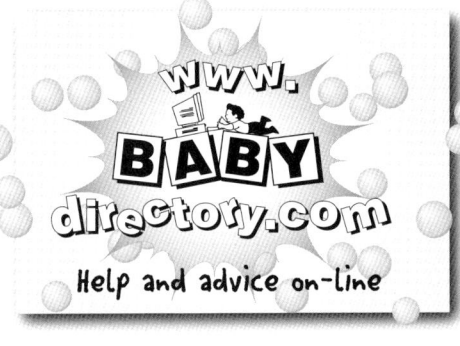

Learn how to massage your baby

Classes for parents and babies

A wonderful way to communicate your love!

Relaxing and fun

Can help relieve colic and improve sleep

For information about local classes Contact:

Carole Barnes C.I.M.I, ITEC
Tel: 020 8979 6261.

International Association of Infant Massage (UK Chapter)

BABY MASSAGE
&
Therapeutic Treatments
Experienced & qualified practitioners

From Bumps to Babies

in our 10th year
Call us for more details on,
Tel: **020 8336 1532**

BABY BLISS
Massage before they crawl

Learn to massage your baby lovingly

Touching and caressing in a loving, caring way is a vital for the physical and emotional well being of your baby. The simple massage techniques learnt will soothe and relax your baby's body, relieving stress and increasing self esteem.
Qualified Baby Massage Tutor
Sarah Spoor
0208 - 568 4913

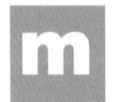

maternity nannies & nurses

(see also doulas, midwives, nanny agencies)

Merstham
TINIES NANNY AGENCY
88 Nutfield Road. 01737 642444
e.surrey@tinieschildcare.co.uk
www.tinieschildcare.co.uk
Most progressive agency with more nannies, maternity nurses, part-time & emergency carers

Cheam
TINIES NANNY AGENCY
Foxhills, 91 Bersford Road
020 8642 2228
n.surrey@tinieschildcare.co.uk
www.tinieschildcare.co.uk
Most progressive agency with more nannies, maternity nurses, part-time & emergency carers

Esher
Mary Ward
01372 469552
Mother/ex-maternity nurse will babysit your new born

Farnborough
TINIES NANNY AGENCY
9 Stanley Drive. 01252 371373
hants@tinieschildcare.co.uk
www.tinieschildcare.co.uk
Most progressive agency with more nannies, maternity nurses, part-time & emergency carers

Richmond
TINIES NANNY AGENCY
210 Parkway House, Sheen Lane
020 8876 4391
richmond@tinieschildcare.co.uk
www.tinieschildcare.co.uk
Most progressive agency with more nannies, maternity nurses, part-time & emergency carers

maternity wear: mail order

BLOOMING MARVELLOUS
020 8391 4822
www.bloomingmarvellous.co.uk

MATERNUS/FORTY WEEKS
020 8299 6761
www.maternus.co.uk
A funky range of maternity basics designed to fit throughout pregnancy

Bumpstart
020 8879 3467

Business Bump
01625 599022

Formes
020 8689 1133

NCT (Maternity Sales) Ltd
239 Shawbridge Street, Glasgow. 0141 636 0600

maternity wear: retail & hire

Mothercare branches in most high streets

Cobham
Blooming Marvellous
23 Oakdene Parade. 01932 864343

Guildford
Formes (UK) Ltd
8 Tunsgate Square. 01483 454777

Kew
MUMS 2 BE
3 Mortlake Terrace, Mortlake Road, Kew, Richmond. 020 8332 6506
For all your fashion needs during pregnancy

mathematics

KUMON EDUCATIONAL
www.kumon.co.uk
0800 854714

Please say you saw the ad in
The Local Baby Directory

www.babydirectory.com   The Local Baby Directory - *Surrey & S. Middlesex*   **Page 55**

maternus
FORTY WEEKS essentials

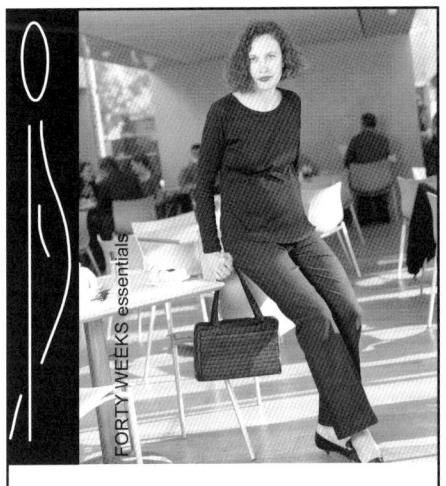

33 Dulwich Village London SE21 7BN
T 020 8299 6761   F 020 8299 6561

Mail Order - Contact us for a free catalogue
or shop online at **www.maternus.co.uk**

Exclusive Spanish & Italian Designs

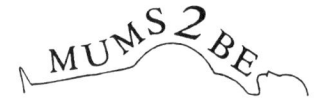

MUMS 2 BE

For all your fashion needs
during pregnancy, from
Business wear to Leisure wear.

Petite Collection available.
Evening Wear Hire.
Bra fitting & Alteration service.

Mon-Sat 10am-5.30pm

⊖ Kew Gardens
Easy parking at rear of shop

3 Mortlake Terrace, Mortlake Road,
Kew, Richmond, Surrey TW9 3DT

020 8332 6506

Established 1992

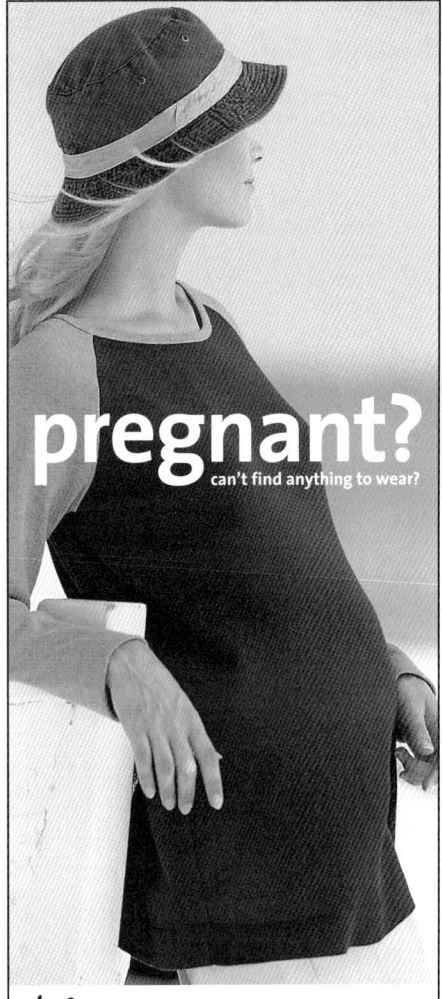

---

pregnant?
can't find anything to wear?

Blooming Marvellous

MUST-HAVE MATERNITY WEAR
ADORABLE BABY CLOTHES   THE CLEVEREST NURSERY IDEAS

For the UK's biggest and best maternity wear catalogue,
call the number below and quote code **BD01**
or visit one of our shops: Bath, Chester, Cobham,
London SW6, St. Albans and Winchester.

020 8391 4822
www.bloomingmarvellous.co.uk

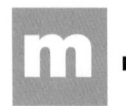

PREGNANT?

Let us provide you with the maternity care *of your dreams*.

* Free initial consultation
* Your personal midwife available 24/7
* Convenient appointments
* Birth at our Birth Centre
* Birth in hospital
* Birth at home
* Privacy
* Active and water births
* Up to six weeks after-care

THE BIRTH CENTRE

Director - Caroline Flint
For Brochure & Information
020 7498 2322

Kingston-upon-Thames
Ginny Ensignia
0958 409514
Active Birth Teacher

Teddington
W. London Independent Midwives
44 Wick Road. 020 8286 7593
wlim@pobox.com
www.netcomuk.co.uk

Tooting
BIRTH CENTRE
37 Coverton Road. 020 8767 8294
www.birthcentre.com

Wraysbury
Southern Counties Midwifery Practice
23 Old School Court. 07711 501577

Yateley
The Borders Birth Practice
32 Lawford Crescent. 01252 409152

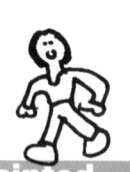

meditation

Calm for Kids
020 8994 5093
calmforkids@aol.com

midwives: independent

(see also antenatal support & information, maternity nannies & nurses)

Independent Midwives' Association
01483 821104

Guildford
Surrey Independent Midwives
1 The Great Quarry. 01483 538615
andrea@dombrowe.globalnet.co.uk

Surrey Independent Midwives
40 Barnett Close, Wonersh. 01483 892525

murals & painted nursery furniture

(see also nursery furniture & decor, nursery goods)

Magical Rooms
020 8893 9448

Mural Magic
01737 555855

Alison Clark
020 8755 0121
pilot3524@aol.com

Kingston-upon-Thames
Stencil Store
Bentalls Shopping Centre, Wood Street
020 8547 3686

Please say you saw the ad in
The Local Baby Directory

museums

(see also outings)

Brentford
Kew Bridge Steam Museum
Green Dragon Lane. 020 8568 4757
Open everyday. Engines only run at weekends, free for under 5's

Musical Museum
368 High Street. 020 8560 8108

Caterham
East Surrey Museum
1 Stafford Road. 01883 340 275
10-5pm Sat, 2-5pm Sun, 10-5pm Wed

Chertsey
Chertsey Museum
The Cedars, 33 Windsor Street. 01932 565 764
Hands on discovery room, time section etc.
12.30-4.30pm Tues.-Fri, 11-4pm Sat

Chichester
Weald & Downland Open Air Museum
Singleton. 01243 811348
www.wealddown.co.uk
40+ historic buildings, working farm and mill, pond with ducks. Children's activity area, picnic area, shop. Special events. Open daily 10.30-6pm (restricted Winter opening times)

Cobham
Cobham Bus Museum
Redhill Road. 01932 868 665
Spring/summer opening

Dorking
Dorking & District Museum
The Old Foundry, 62a West Street
01306 876 591

Farnham
Museum Of Farnham
West Street. 01252 715 094
10-5pm Tues-Sat

Rural Life Centre
Old Kiln Museum, The Reeds, Tilford
01252 792 300
Spring/summer opening

Godalming
Godalming Museum
109a High Street. 01483 426 510
10-4pm Tues-Sat

Guildford
Guildford Museum
Castle Arch, Quarry Street. 01483 444 750
Victorian toys etc, 11-5pm except Sun

Haslemere
Haslemere Educational Museum
78 High Street. 01428 642 112

Kingston-upon-Thames
Kingston Museum & Heritage Service
Wheatfield Way. 020 8546 5386
10-5pm Mon, Tues, Thurs, Fri, Sat

Mitcham
Merton Heritage Centre
The Cannons, Madeira Road. 020 8640 9387
10-5pm Fri & Sat

Mitcham
Wandle Industrial Museum
Vestry Hall Annex, London Road
020 8648 0127
1-4pm Wed plus 1st Sun of the month 2-5pm

Reigate
Reigate Priory Museum
Reigate Priory, Bell Street. 01737 222550

Richmond
Museum of Richmond
Old Town Hall, Whittaker Avenue
020 8332 1141
11-5pm Tues-Sat

Weybridge
Elmbridge Museum
Church Street. 01932 843 573
Children's activity area, closed Thurs & Sun,
11-5pm weekdays, 10-1pm, 2-5pm Sat

Visit us at
www.babydirectory.com

music

(see also art, dance, drama)

MONKEY MUSIC
01582 766464
www.monkeymusic.co.uk
Action songs and rhymes, music and movement, fun with percussion and musical games

MUSICAL MINIS
020 8329 8620
www.musicalminis.co.uk
Northeast Surrey. The fun time music group for babies & toddlers

NATIONAL FOUNDATION FOR YOUTH MUSIC
One America Street, London SE1
020 7902 1060
www.youthmusic.org.uk
Funding and music projects for prenatal babies - five-year olds

Andrew Rankin
01825 790478
Violin lessons 2yrs+

Le Kinder Club
020 8943 5363
Up to 5yrs

Little Acorns Nursery Music Workshops
020 8408 0322
1-3yrs. Banstead, Carshalton & Cheam

Mini Minstrels
0845 345 5550

Musical Playtime
01372 378651
charyl@musical-playtime.co.uk
Fetcham, Bookham, Stoke d'Abernon & Tadworth

Noahs Ark Music Club
020 8941 8377
Molesey, Claygate, Hersham & Ewell

Polka Dots
01932 571311
18mths-3yrs. Walton & Weybridge

Music classes for babies and young children!

Monkey Music introduces music to very young children in a way they can easily understand and enjoy. Since 1992, thousands of children have participated with specialist teachers in local classes across London and the South East. Classes are arranged in three levels, according to age, from 6 months to 4 years.

Call to book a FREE introductory session today!

For classes in your area, please call the
Central Reservation Line
01582 766464
www.monkeymusic.co.uk

Try a Monkey Music Party

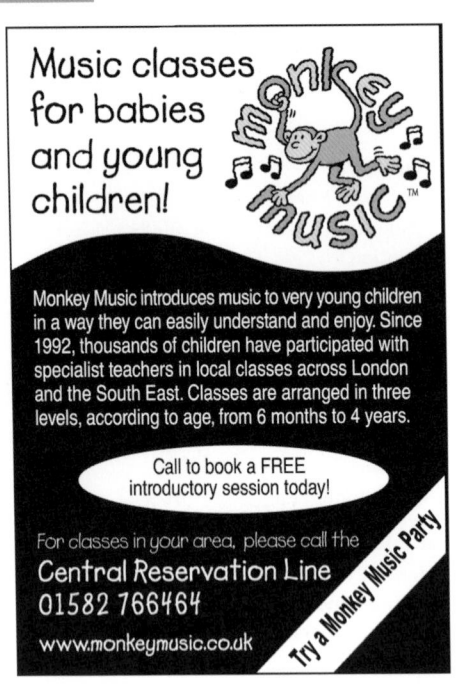

FIRST STEPS

Babies and toddlers can take their First Steps into music making with the help of Youth Music funding and projects. Parents and early years specialists can also benefit from music training.

To find out more about the programme visit:
www.youthmusic.org.uk
or call 08450 560 560

Funded by the Arts Council of England

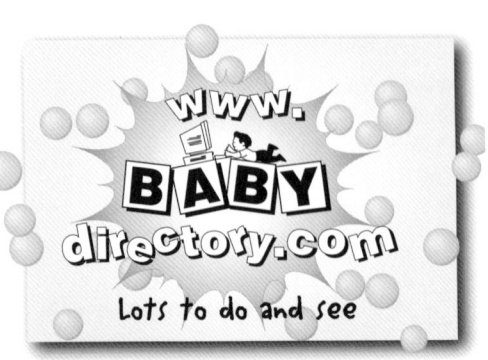

national foundation for youth music

---

www.BABYdirectory.com
Lots to do and see

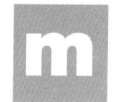

Silverball Kids
020 8384 4417
Hounslow, Twickenham, Teddington,
Whitton. Under 5's

Camberley
Kindermusik
01276 62407
www.kindermusik.com
0-7yrs

Caterham
jo jingles
01883 712881

Cobham
Buttons & Bows
01932 866595

Farnham
jo jingles
01252 794329

Feltham
Hounslow Schools Music Service
Debrome Building, Boundaries Road
020 583 2000

Guildford
Music with Mummy
01483 833780

Hampton
Music Time
020 8979 8923
Under 5's

Oxted
jo jingles
01883 712881

Redhill
jo jingles
01883 712881

Reigate
jo jingles
01883 712881

Richmond
BLUEBERRY PLAYSONGS
Queen of Peace Church Hall,
222 Sheen Road. 020 8677 6871
blueberry@clara.co.uk
www.blueberry.clara.co.uk
9mths-4yrs

Centres: Clapham · Putney · Chelsea · Hammersmith
Richmond · Notting Hill · Barnes · Wimbledon

learning to have fun with music
for ages 9 months - 4 years

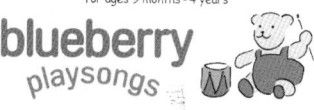

blueberry
playsongs

Guitar accompanied action songs, nursery rhymes, instruments,
games & dancing - come and try the blueberry experience!
www.blueberry.clara.co.uk • blueberry@clara.co.uk

Call: 020 8677 6871

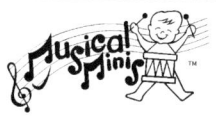

THE FUN TIME MUSIC GROUP FOR
BABIES & TODDLERS FROM 6 MONTHS +
Introducing music and percussion in a relaxed
group atmosphere.
GROUPS LOCALLY
Telephone: Sarah on 020 8239 8620
(Established 1990)

Colourstrings
020 8948 2066
6mths-5yrs

Mini Maestro's
020 8783 0436

Sutton
Music Land
020 8773 8863

Twickenham
Tuneful Toddlers
Etna Community Centre, 13 Rosslyn Road
020 8892 1355
1-3yrs. Thurs/Fri am

Walton-on-Thames
Little Mozarts
01932 226991
1-4yrs

Please say you saw the ad in
The Local Baby Directory

Off to Nursery? Use EASY2NAME

* Dishwasher proof stickers
* Iron-on tapes and transfers
* You name it - we label it!

For samples phone - 01635-298326

www.easy2name.com

name tapes

EASY2NAME
01635 298326
easy2name@aol.com
www.easy2name.com
Easy2name suppliers of dishwasher proof stickers and iron-on tapes

SIMPLY STUCK
01264 350788
www.simplystuck.com
Innovative personalised name labels. Tested by thousands of children!

Welcome to The World!
Baby Naming Ceremonies

Acknowledge the gift of new life.... Many parents are asking for help in arranging a 'special' ceremony to welcome their new child.
Naming ceremonies are a secular alternative, each is written individually and can be conducted for you by an Accredited Celebrant. These are wonderful, warm and joyous occasions; a time to gather family and friends; to pledge your love and commitment, joy and hopes for your child's future and to formally give their name.

For more details, please call Vivienne on
01932 862116
www.ceremony.org.uk

naming ceremonies

(see also registration of births)

ALTERNATIVE CEREMONIES
01932 862116

Baby Naming Society
Yeoman's Cottage, Kerswell Green, Kempsey, Worcestershire. 01905 371070

British Humanist Association
47 Theobald's Road, London WC1
020 7430 0908
National Helpline 0990 168122

www.babydirectory.com

We have a Nanny Agency On-line

nanny agencies

(see also au pair agencies, babysitters, childcare listings magazine, childminders, maternity nannies & nurses)

MONTROSE AGENCY INTERNATIONAL
23 Bullescroft Road, Edgware, Middx
020 8958 9209
montrose@taylor.clara.net
We listen, we care, we make the right connections. Established 22 years

MONTROSE AGENCY INTERNATIONAL
Mothers Helps / Nannies / Au-Pairs

We listen, we care, we make the right connections.

Call **Linda** or **Barbra** for a personal, friendly service.

e-mail: montrose@taylor.clara.net

TEL: 020 8958-9209

Night Nannies
Sevenacres, Church Hill, Binfield, Berkshire, RG42 5PY

Does your baby need feeding at night?

Has your child got sleep problems?

Are you longing for a good night out and lie-in the following day?

"Get yourself a good night's sleep"
and call on our team of experienced Night Nannies.

Tel: 01344 862 973
Email: iona@night-nannies.com

Nannies/nurses in Surrey with newborn experience needed to work nights to help parents.

Wimbledon Nannies

Temporary and Permanent work, both Daily and Residential, Full and Part time. All staff interviewed and checked. Evening Babysitting Register

Established 1985   REC member
020 8947 4666
fax: 020 8947 0405
e-mail: info@wimbledonnannies.co.uk   www.wimbledonnannies.com
184 Copse Hill, Wimbledon SW20 0SP

Nanny Service
6 Nottingham Street, London W1
020 7935 3515

Needananny
0800 956 1212
www.needananny.net
Providing quality childcare to private families

NIGHT NANNIES
01344 862973
iona@night-nannies.com

WIMBLEDON NANNIES
184 Copse Hill, London, SW20
020 8947 4666
info@wimbledonnannies.com
www.wimbledonnannies.co.uk
For a professional and friendly service look no further

Tinies
Childcare for the modern world

With 25 years experience, a childcare agency for today's Parents and Carers

- **Nannies**
- **Maternity Nannies**
- **Mothers Helps**

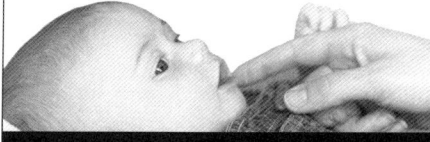

For your nearest branch call
0800 783 6070
www.tinies.co.uk

Please say you saw the ad in
The Local Baby Directory

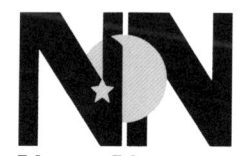

KEW Nannies
In Safe Hands

- Full/part-time nannies •
- Mother's helps •
- Maternity nurses •
- Baby-sitting register •

020 8332 0944

Home visits with no obligation
All staff interviewed and checked

• Kew Nannies Ltd • 20 Priory Road • Kew •
• Surrey • London • TW9 3DF •
Tel + Fax: 020 8332 0944

www.kewnannies.com

STRAWBERRY HILL NANNIES

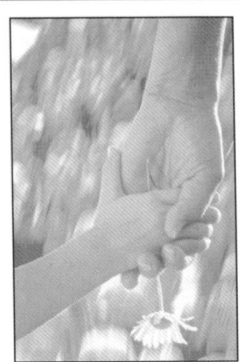

"Helping children to dream with their eyes open"

- Nannies and Mother's Helps
- Babysitting Service
- All Clients and Nannies personally interviewed face to face

TEL: 020 8891 0911

HOME Away From HOME
International Childcare

❖ Au Pairs
❖ Nannies
❖ Parents' Help
❖ After school pickup/care
❖ Babysitters
❖ Domestics

All carers have references and are fully vetted
Au pairs available from most
EC/non-EC countries
(National coverage)
For your Childcare Needs Call:

Tel: 020 8763 1206
Fax: 020 8405 0678
Mobile: 07764 341777

Email: homeawayfromhome@bigfoot.com
www.homeawayfromhomechildcare.co.uk

---

the Nanny agency

We ...
• meet you and <u>all</u> our nannies and mothers helps

• check our nannies refs and qualifications

• offer you advice and guidance

• provide a follow up service

<u>We provide full or part time nannies, mothers helps, babysitters etc.</u>

Walton on Thames, Surrey

01932 240323
Email:
surrey@thenanny agency.co.uk

Select Nannies

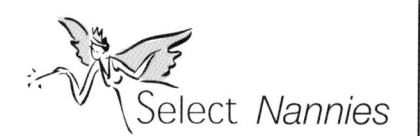

Select Nannies is THE professional nanny service for the Surrey area.

We:
- Meet and interview ALL nannies and families
- Check references and qualifications
- Ensure all nannies are police checked
- Fit the right nanny to the right family
- Offer continued advice and guidance

And we can suit your needs whether full or part-time, live-in or daily.

We know how important your child is and we offer only the best people and service.

For further details call Angela Spencer on
01932 402146

nanny agencies (cont.)

Cheam
TINIES NANNY AGENCY
Foxhills, 91 Bersford Road. 020 8642 8866
n.surrey@tinieschildcare.co.uk
www.tinieschildcare.co.uk
Most progressive agency with more nannies, maternity nurses, part-time & emergency carers

Farnborough
TINIES NANNY AGENCY
9 Stanley Drive. 01252 371373
hants@tinieschildcare.co.uk
www.tinieschildcare.co.uk
Most progressive agency with more nannies, maternity nurses, part-time & emergency carers

Kew
KEW NANNIES
20 Priory Road. 020 8332 0944
www.kewnannies.com

Merstham
TINIES NANNY AGENCY
88 Nutfield Road. 01737 642444
e.surrey@tinieschildcare.co.uk
www.tinieschildcare.co.uk
Most progressive agency with more nannies, maternity nurses, part-time & emergency carers

Purley
HOME AWAY FROM HOME
10 Hartley Down. 020 8763 1206

Putney
NANNIES UNLIMITED
11 Chelverton Road. 020 8788 9640
enquiries@nanniesunlimited.co.uk
www.nanniesunlimited.co.uk
The professional and caring agency for both nannies and families

Richmond
TINIES NANNY AGENCY
210 Parkway House. 020 8876 4391
richmond@tinieschildcare.co.uk
www.tinieschildcare.co.uk
Most progressive agency with more nannies, maternity nurses, part-time & emergency carers

Strawberry Hill
STRAWBERRY HILL NANNIES
9 Waldegrave Gardens. 020 8891 0911

Twickenham
JUST IN THE BOX NANNIES LTD
020 8241 4178
jackintheboxnannies@yahoo.co.uk
Agency offering quality childcare to suit every individual, covering local areas

Walton-on-Thames
THE NANNY AGENCY
25 Station Avenue. 01932 240323
surrey@thenannyagency.co.uk
www.thenannyagency.co.uk

West Byfleet
SELECT NANNIES
01932 402146

Please say you saw the ad in
The Local Baby Directory

Nanny Payroll Service

Everything necessary is done to pay your nanny correctly

We advise and implement nanny shares

Nationwide service

Fees £110 pa (incl VAT)

The Studio Benefield Road Brigstock NN14 3ES

Tel: 01536 373111
Fax 01536 373123

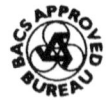

BACS APPROVED BUREAU

www.nannypayroll.co.uk

nanny payroll services

(see also financial advice)

NANNYTAX
PO Box 988, Brighton BN2 1BY
01273 626256
mailbox@nannytax.co.uk
www.nannytax.co.uk
Nannytax is the UK's leading payroll service for parents employing a nanny

NANNY PAYROLL SERVICE
Payday Services Ltd,
The Studio, Benefield Road, Brigstock,
Kettering, Northants
01536 373111
www.nannypayroll.co.uk

Please say you saw the ad in **The Local Baby Directory**

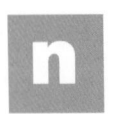

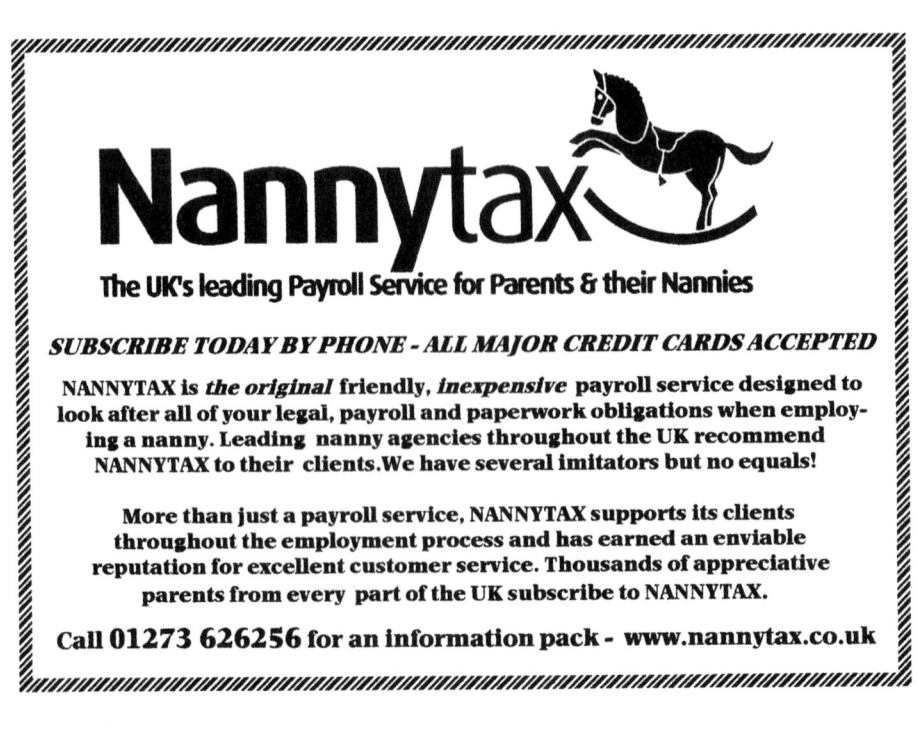

Nannytax

The UK's leading Payroll Service for Parents & their Nannies

SUBSCRIBE TODAY BY PHONE - ALL MAJOR CREDIT CARDS ACCEPTED

NANNYTAX is *the original* friendly, *inexpensive* payroll service designed to look after all of your legal, payroll and paperwork obligations when employing a nanny. Leading nanny agencies throughout the UK recommend NANNYTAX to their clients. We have several imitators but no equals!

More than just a payroll service, NANNYTAX supports its clients throughout the employment process and has earned an enviable reputation for excellent customer service. Thousands of appreciative parents from every part of the UK subscribe to NANNYTAX.

Call 01273 626256 for an information pack - www.nannytax.co.uk

nappies: cloth & other

BABY BLISS
020 8568 4913

Bambino Mio
01604 883777

Bonny Baby Company
01428 683722
www.bonnybabyco.com

Cotton Bottoms
01798 875300

Kooshies
31-33 Park Royal Road, London, NW10
0870 607 0545
www.thebabycatalogue.com
Kooshies washable nappies and all baby products in a mail order catalogue

Plush Pants Cloth Nappies
55 Newlands Avenue, Cheadle Hulme, Cheshire. 0161 485 4430
www.plushpants.co.uk
Nappies, wraps, accessories, baby clothes and treats for mum too

Spirit of Nature Ltd
01582 847370

West London Real Nappy Campaign "Nappy Night"

Find out about real nappies, nappy services and home washing. Come to a "Nappy Night". Held on the 2nd Tuesday of every month. Look at the various real nappies on the market and discover what will work for you, your baby and your lifestyle. All aspects of nappy use covered, environmental cost, financial cost and health implications.

Sarah Spoor - 0208 568 4913

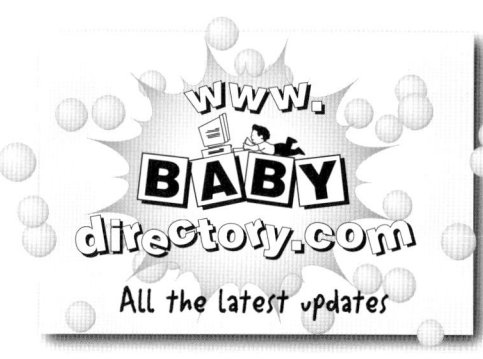

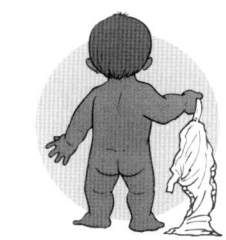

---

nappy information

National Association of Nappy Services (NANS)
01021 6934949
Find out where your nearest nappy laundry laundry service is.
www.changeanappy.co.uk

Real Nappy Association
PO Box 3704, London, SE26 4RX. 020 8299 4519
Information on all nappy-related issues

WEST LONDON REAL NAPPY NIGHTS
020 8568 4913

Womens Environmental Network
020 7481 9004
www.nappies@wen.org.uk

nappy delivery & laundry

National Association of Nappy Services (NANS)
01021 6934949
Find out where your nearest nappy laundry laundry service is.
www.changeanappy.co.uk

Nappycare
020 8998 8799

Number 1s for Nappies
271 Holdbrook Court, Holdbrook South
020 8351 0101

Aloe Vera contains over 200 active ingredients, and is the principal component in our unique range of top quality drinking gels, hair & skin care products, supplements, and beehive products with a 90 day money-back guarantee.

For an info pack call
020 8608 1857.

mum and me

Specialising in nearly new baby equipment, toys and clothes from birth to 12 years.

Now in BIGGER premises at
61 High Street, Teddington, Middlesex

There is a LARGER range of everything we've been selling successfully for the last 7 years & MORE SPACE to see it in.

Rental of baby equipment available.
New fancy dress clothes sold at great prices.

For more information call Angela/Anne on
020 8255 0073
Opening Hours:
Mon-Fri 9.30am-4.00pm/Sat 9.30am-5.30pm
(Later by appointment)

natural products

(see also complementary health, organics)

ALOE VERA HEALTH & BEAUTY
020 8608 1857
kateandchris@blueyonder.co.uk

THE KEEPER
020 8608 1857
kateandchris@blueyonder.co.uk
Reusable sanitary protection. Unique product, environmental, convenient, economical. 90 day money-back guarentee

nearly new equipment, toy & clothing shops

Addlestone
Pixies
5 The Broadway. 01932 349864

Feltham
Trading Places
112 The Centre. 020 8893 2960

Gomshall
Kids Swop Shop
Gomshall Lodge East. 01483 298875
Thurs 10-4pm

Surbiton
Rascals
127 Ewell Road. 020 8286 1111

Teddington
MUM AND ME
61 High Street. 020 8255 0073

Walton-on-Thames
Poppy's Children's Centre
119a Hersham Road. 01932 221121

West Byfleet
Little Shop for Horrors
108b High Road. 01932 341119

Weybridge
Bambini
27 Church Street. 01932 857665

nurseries: private & nursery schools

(see also education, schools, tuition)

There is an overlap in the field of private childcare provision and education, and many of the terms seem to be interchangeable amongst the providers. These listings include the full gamut, from nurseries to Montessori nurseries, day nurseries and nursery schools. **Pre-prep schools** (preparing the child for big school, usually at seven years old) have been listed under the schools section, though they often have a nursery class for three or four year olds, and this section should also be consulted. **Prep school** then takes your child through to eleven or thirteen by which time you will have well outgrown this book *(see family planning).*

Babies from three months onwards can attend a **nursery**, and where a full day's care is offered (eg. 8am-6pm) we have tried to indicate this in the notes. In many of these nurseries, older children will graduate from the baby section to a more structured section very like a nursery school, but with longer hours for play, sleep, etc. In general, a **crèche** only offers a few hours of unstructured supervision, while parents do something else *(see drop-in nurseries, health clubs with crèches, shopping crèches).* At a **playgroup** *(qv)* the carer usually remains in attendance. A **nursery school** for $2^1/2$ to five year olds usually follows a basic school day (9am-3.30pm) and term but pupils may attend only one session, morning or afternoon. Many nurseries use **Montessori** methods, a system devised by Maria Montessori in 1907 which emphasises training of the senses and encouragement rather than a rigid academic curriculum.

For nearly all nurseries and schools in the private sector, early registration is recommended, so ring, visit and inform yourself in time, even if you later decide not to pursue that option.

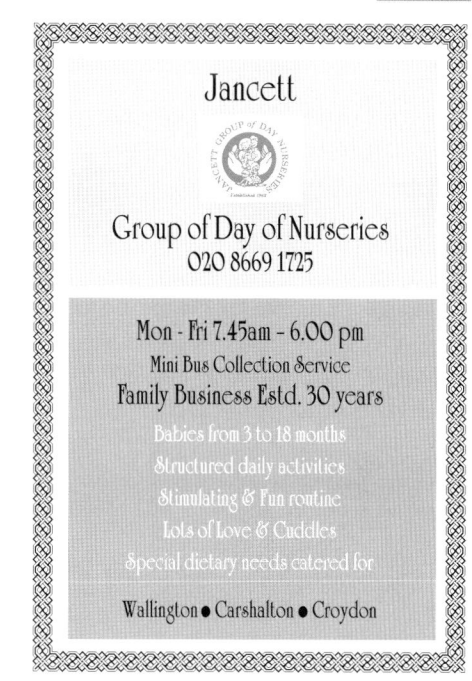

Jancett

Group of Day of Nurseries
020 8669 1725

Mon - Fri 7.45am - 6.00 pm
Mini Bus Collection Service
Family Business Estd. 30 years

Babies from 3 to 18 months
Structured daily activities
Stimulating & Fun routine
Lots of Love & Cuddles
Special dietary needs catered for

Wallington • Carshalton • Croydon

For a list of **state-run** nurseries, or state primary schools with nursery classes attached, contact your Under 8s section at the local council *(see under councils)* or check out www.childcare.gov.uk or Childcare Link on 08000 96 02 96. Good luck! You'll need it.

JANCETT GROUP OF DAY NURSERIES
020 8669 1725
admin@jancett.co.uk

TEDDIES NURSERIES
020 8744 1531
See advert on page 69

Addlestone
Buckles & Bows Pre-school Nursery
Holy Family RC Primary School. 01932 827556
$2^1/2$-5yrs

Please say you saw the ad in
The Local Baby Directory

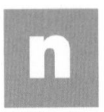

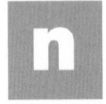

**ST DAVID'S JUNIOR SCHOOL
& DRAGON PARK NURSERY**
Church Road, Ashford, Middx, TW15 3DZ

Come and see us!

Telephone 01784 252494 for details

---

nurseries: private & nursery schools (cont.)

Farthings Nursery School
Church Road. 01932 840179
2½-5yrs

St George's College Junior School
Weybridge Road. 01932 839300
www.st-georges-college.co.uk

Teddies on a Rainbow
Heathervale Pavillion. 01932 352516
2½-5yrs

Ash Vale
Cherryvale Nursery
Frimley Road. 01252 545477

Ashford
DRAGON PARK NURSERY SCHOOL
St David's Junior School. 01784 252494

Fledglings Montessori Nursery School
Spelthorne College. 01784 246578

Patchwork Pieces Nursery School
Ashford High School. 01784 252855
2-5yrs

Ashtead
Flying Start day Nursery
Barnsmead. 01372 276825
3mths-5yrs

Bagshot
Bagshot Community Pre-school
The Pavillion. 01276 452623
2-5yrs

Banstead
Burgh Wood Montessori Nursey School
St Anns Church Hall. 01737 356105
2½- 5yrs

The Old Barn Day Nursery
6 Woodmansterne Lane. 01737 373715

Brentford
Bringing up Baby, Brentford Day Nursery
Half Acre. 020 8568 7561
3mths-5yrs

Buttercups Nurseries
The Garden House. 020 8568 4355
3mths-5yrs

Just Kidding
44 Boston Park Road. 020 8568 4447

Ladybird Lane Day Nursery
St Faiths Church Hall. 020 8232 8839
2-5yrs

Mereleigh Tots Day Nursery
126 Ealing Road. 020 8568 2364
2-5yrs

TEDDIES NURSERIES
The Old School Building. 020 8847 3799
3mths-5yrs
See advert on page 69

Byfleet
YELLOW SUBMARINE PRE-SCHOOL
Methodist Church, Rectory Lane
01932 402593
rshepburn@ntlworld.com
www.childcarelink.gov.uk
Providing a caring environment where children learn best through play

Camberley
Blackberries Creche
Newfoundland Road. 01252 837128

Blackdown Preschool
Blackdown Primary School. 01252 834685
2½-5yrs

www.babydirectory.com The Local Baby Directory - *Surrey & S. Middlesex* **Page 69**

TEDDIES NURSERIES

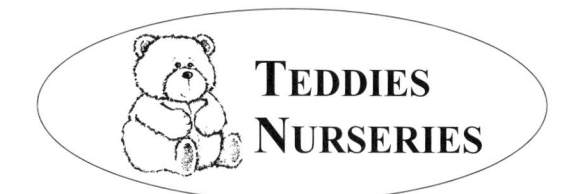

We pride ourselves on giving your child only the very best.

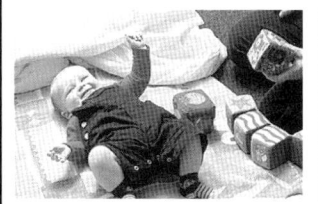

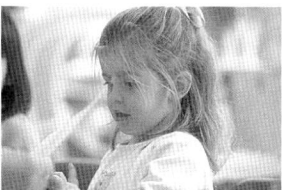

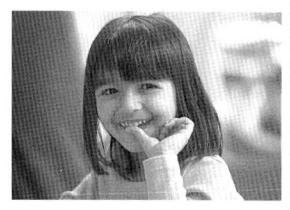

Teddies is one of the UK's leading childcare providers, providing care for children from three months to five years.

Care is available 51 weeks a year, 8pm-6pm Mon-Fri.

- Introduce your child to a whole new world of learning
- Come and see the safe, fun and stimulating environment of our excellent nursery
- Meet our qualified, experienced and caring staff
- We offer full time and part time care (including half days)

Godalming, Esher, Farnham, Woking, Sutton, Croydon

Greenwich, Loughton, Crawley, Bracknell/Ascot,
Newbury, Streatham, Balham, Southfields, Twickenham, Brentford,
Chiswick, Barnes, Northwood, West Hampstead.

For more information call
0800 980 3801
www.teddiesnurseries.co.uk

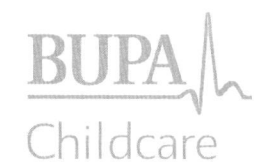

BUPA Childcare

nurseries: private & nursery schools (cont.)

Crawley Ridge Nursery
Crawley County First School. 01276 676158
2¹/₂-5yrs

Elands Day Nursery
49 Park Road. 01276 22582
2-5yrs

Hatton Hill Day Nursery
1 The Green, Frimley Green. 01252 838638
3mths-5yrs

The Nursery School
1 The Green. 01252 835123
2-4yrs

St Pauls Nursery
St Pauls Church Hall. 01276 22881

Carshalton
Carshalton Methodist Day Nursery
Ruskin Road. 020 8669 3676

Springboard Kindergarten
39 Street Andrews Road. 020 8395 5050

Caterham
Asquith Court Nursery
Burntwood Lane. 01883 341988

Caterham Pre-School & Nursery
Burntwood Lane. 01883 330122

Charlwood
CRANBROOK
(THE FARMHOUSE) LTD
Horley Road. 01293 823279
0-3yrs
See advert on page 77

CRANBROOK NURSERY SCHOOL
The Farmhouse, Horley Road
01293 823279
0-3yrs
See advert on page 77

Cheam
Nonsuch Park Montessori School
The Lodge, Nonsuch Park. 020 8393 2419
2¹/₂-5yrs

Chertsey
Cherry Nursery
Staines Lane. 01932 570580

Rainbow Nursery
Pyrcroft Road. 01932 570775

Chessington
Microtots Nursery
Chessington Computer Centre. 020 8391 3330
3mths-5yrs

Moor Lane Workplace Nursery
Moor Lane. 020 8391 2113
3mths-5yrs

Playtime Day Nursery
Church Rise. 020 8397 2800
3mths-5yrs

Chiswick
DEVONSHIRE DAY NURSERY
(CHILD BASE)
Bennett Street, W4 2AH. 020 8995 9538
devonshire@childbase.com
www.childbase.com
We Care As Much As You

Cobham
Fairmile Montessori School
Cobham Rugby Club. 01372 469500
2-5yrs

Coulsdon
Hillcrest Montessori Nursery School
Hillcrest Hall. 020 8763 6284
2¹/₂-5yrs

The Mulberry Bush Pre-School
The Scout Hut. 020 8660 4180
2¹/₂-4yrs

Cranleigh
Christopher Robin Day Nursery
Christopher Robin House. 01483 277050

Cranleigh Nursery School
Fair View. 01483 274693
2¹/₂-5yrs

Visit us at
www.babydirectory.com

The Little School (Montessori)
Loxworth Road. 01403 752350

Croydon
Croydon Playcare Co
Gingerbread Corner. 020 8684 8848

Early Learners
26 Church Road. 020 8681 8430
6wks-5yrs

Early Learners
rear of 62 High Street. 020 8688 2161
6wks-5yrs

Indigo House Montessori Nursery School
30 Northampton Road. 020 8655 4545

Little Gems Day Nursery
9 Heathfield Road. 020 8667 1345

Saplings Day Nursery
48 Sydenham Road. 020 8681 7579
3mths-5yrs

TEDDIES NURSERIES
Esporta Health Club. 020 8253 1320
See advert on page 69

Tender Care Nursery
32 Oakfield Road. 020 8681 6263

Thornton Heath Early Years Centre
Nursery Road. 020 8684 0494
2-5yrs

Dorking
Amicus Day Nursery Ltd
Nutcombe House. 01306 880842

Chatterbox Nursery
The Ashcombe School. 01306 742050

East Molesey
Rosalita Edwards Montessori Nursery & Daycare
East Molesey Cricket Club. 020 8979 2542
2-5yrs

Egham
Englefield Green Montessori School
Kings Lane. 01784 472668
2½-5yrs

Little Echoes Day Nursery School
The Orchard. 01784 433279

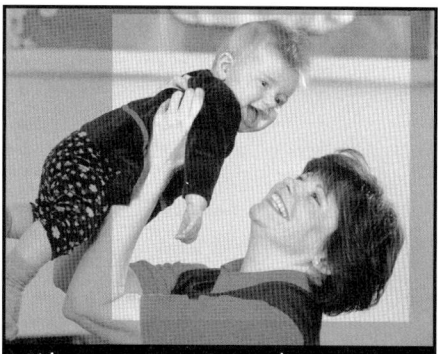

We care as much as you

Think of Child Base as a home from home. Where your child will receive the same loving care and attention and play happily with other children of the same age. Giving you more time for your busy lifestyle.

Child Base operates over 30 nurseries, each to the same high standard of care. With a highly qualified, motivated team of nursery nurses, whose only interest is in creating a stimulating environment and caring for your child.

- 6 weeks to 5 years old
- Full time places or sessions
- Highly trained, caring staff

For a prospectus and further details please call:

Knowle Green Day Nursery
Knowle Green, Staines TW18 1AJ
Tel: 01784 464141

Devonshire Day Nursery
Bennett Street, Chiswick W4 2AH
Tel: 020 8995 9538

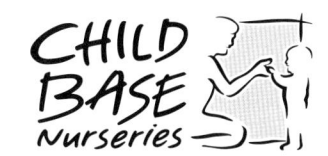

CHILD BASE Nurseries
Care and Early Teaching Centres
www.childbase.com

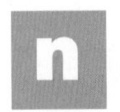

nurseries: private & nursery schools (cont.)

Mancroft Nursery
Wesley Drive. 01784 438977
2¹/2-5yrs

Milton Hall Montessori School
Social Hall, Harvest Road. 01784 471572
2¹/2-5yrs

Epsom

Asquith Court Nursery
28 Worple Road. 01372 723322

Concorde Nursery
Concorde Scout Hall, The Footpath
01372 742502
3-5yrs

Cunliffe Day Nursery
Cunliffe House, Cunliffe Road. 020 786 8921
2-5yrs

Epsom Christian Fellowship Playgroup
Cornerstone School, 22-24 West Hill
01372 742940

Epsom Methodist Nursery
Epsom Methodist Church, Ashley Road
01372 727915
3-5yrs

Epsom Playhouse Pre-School
Epsom Playhouse, Ashley Ave. 01372 742555
3-5yrs

Ferndale Nursery
St Martins Scout Hall, Church Road
01372 726193
2-5yrs

Gatehouse Nursery
28 Worple Road. 01372 723322
3mths-5yrs

The Kindergarten
St John's Chandler Hall. 01372 726902

Little Group
St Josephs School. 01372 720218
Special needs

Little Hands Nursery
Christchurch Scout HQ. 01372 729986
2-5yrs

PETITS ENFANTS DAY NURSERY
St Ebbas Hospital. 01372 749778
3mths-5yrs

The Railway Children Kindergarten
Station House. 01372 802549
2¹/2-5yrs

St Barnabas Nursery
Hook Road. 020 642 1175
2-5yrs

St Martins Pre School
Church House, Church Street. 01372 722567
2¹/2-5yrs

Time for Tots Daycare & PreSchool Nursery
The Old Dairy, 1 Dell Lane. 020 8786 8006
3mths-5yrs

The Wells Road Pre School
Spa Drive. 01372 724614
2¹/2-5yrs

Esher

Claygate Montessori
Church Road. 01372 844368

Hatton Hill Nursery
01372 473970
3mths-5yrs

TEDDIES NURSERIES
5 Wolsey Road. 01372 210904
See advert on page 69

Ewell

St Clements Nursery School
St Clements Church Hall, 307 Kingston Road
020 8393 5572
2¹/2-5yrs

The Oaks Kindergarten
United Reform Church Hall, London Road
020 8393 0866
3-5yrs

Please say you saw the ad in
The Local Baby Directory

petits enfants

DAY NURSERIES

Cheam, Epsom, Fulham, Fulwell, Morden, Sth Wimbledon, Teddington, Thames Ditton, Sutton

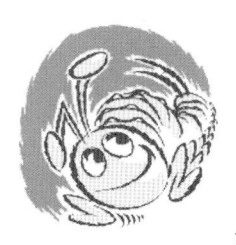

☆ A safe, happy & caring environment

☆ Child friendly gardens

☆ Enthusiastic, qualified staff

☆ Unique sensory areas

☆ Pre-school for 2-5's

☆ Computer & technology facilities

☆ 3 mths - 5 yrs, full or part-time sessions

☆ 7.30am to 6pm, Mon-Fri throughout the year

Call (020) 8977 0333
E-mail sharoma@church-road.fslife.co.uk
for further information
or visit our website:
www.petits-enfants.co.uk

Petits Enfants Day Nurseries Ltd.   Registered No. 2983842

INVESTOR IN PEOPLE

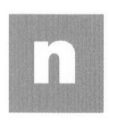

The Little Pegasus Nursery

at

CLEWBOROUGH HOUSE SCHOOL at CHESWYCKS,
Frimley Green, Surrey

for children aged from 2 years

The Little Pegasus Nursery aims to provide a happy and stimulating atmosphere in which the intellectual, physical, emotional and social development of very young children can be promoted under close and caring supervision.

For more information or to arrange a visit please contact us:
Tel: 01252 835669 or 01276 24799 Fax: 01276 24424
Email: head@clewbrgh.demon.co.uk
or visit the school's website at www.clewbrgh.demon.co.uk
GUILDFORD ROAD, FRIMLEY GREEN, SURREY, GU16 6PB

---

nurseries: private & nursery schools (cont.)

Farnham
Farnham Nursery School
Monks Walk. 01252 714286

First Child Care
40 Frensham Vale. 01252 795800

TEDDIES NURSERIES
4 Cambridge Place. 01252 721268
3mths-5yrs
See advert on page 69

Feltham
Once Upon a Time Nursery
Sea Cadet Hall, Poplar Way. 020 751 5810
18mths-5yrs

St George's Early Learning Nursery School
St George's Church Hall. 020 8831 9980
2-5yrs

Frimley Green
LITTLE PEGASUS NURSERY
Clewborough House School at Cheswycks. 01252 835669
head@clewbrgh.demon.co.uk

Godalming
Hollies Nursery School
Thursley Village Hall. 01252 703835
2^1/$_2$-5yrs

Godalming
Little Acorns Nursery School
The Barn, Penang Farm. 01428 685633
2-5yrs, plus holiday & after school clubs

Rainbows Nursery School
The Village Hall. 01252 703414
2^1/$_2$-5yrs

Rocking Horse Nursery
7 Woodside Park. 01483 860273
3mths-5yrs

TEDDIES NURSERIES
0800 980 3801
www.teddiesnurseries.co.uk
See advert on page 69

Tuesley Nursery School
Petworth Road. 01483 861904
2-5yrs

The Wharf Nursery School
The Wharf. 01483 415220

Witley Montessori School
Chichester Hall. 01428 685463

Guildford
Asquith Court Nursery
56 Epsom Road. 01483 578569

Burpham Pre-School
Church of the Holy Spirit. 01483 302635
2^1/$_2$-5yrs

CASTLE NURSERY
14 South Hill. 01483 533344
castle@daycare.co.uk
6mths-5yrs
See advert on page 75

CASTLE NURSERY AT SHAMLEY GREEN
Guildford Road. 01483 898811
info@daycare.co.uk

CASTLE NURSERY AT SPECTRUM
Guildford Spectrum. 01483 443358
spectrum@daycare.co.uk

Christopher Robin Day Nursery
Christpher Robin House. 01483 303474

The Dene Nursery School
The Dene. 01483 561652

Emmanuel Church Nursery
Glaziers Lane. 01483 810683
2 1/2-5yrs

Fitzsimmons Place Nursery
32 Portsmouth Road. 01483 455133
3mths-5yrs

Guildford Pre-School & Nursery
56 Epsom Road. 01483 440299
3mths-5yrs

Shepherds Hill Nursery School
Worplesdon Road. 01483 562550

Shere Montessori Nursery School
Gomshall Lane. 01483 202715
6mths-5yrs

The Wonersh Nursery School
Wonersh Memorial Hall. 01483 898787

Halliford Village
Chestnuts Nursery School
Halliford Community Centre. 01932 82260

Hampton
Asquith Court Nursery
30 Station Road. 020 8979 2098

ASTON PIERPOINT NURSERY & PRE-SCHOOL
34 Priory Road. 0870 046 3301
info@astonpierpont.com
www.astonpierpoint.com
Leading the way in childcare & education
0-5yrs

Grassroots Nursery School
24 Ashley Road. 020 8783 1190
3mths-5yrs

Greenacres
68 Priory Road. 020 8941 1493
3mths-5yrs

Castle Childcare

We are dedicated to encouraging a sense of curiosity in all children in our care. In a stimulating environment with gentle guidance from qualified staff, we provide a secure place for children to develop educationally and socially, and enjoy themselves in the process.

We offer full day childcare and nursery education from 8am to 6pm all year round for children from the ages of 3 months to 5 years

We have 3 daycare centres in the Guildford area

Guildford Town Centre close to the High Street	01483 533344
Spectrum Leisure Centre great for A3 & Park & Ride	01483 443358
Shamley Green in a quiet rural location	01483 898811

Email: info@daycare.co.uk
www.daycare.co.uk

---

aston pierpoint

New Nursery & Pre School
In Priory Road, Hampton

- **We Care**
  Your Childs needs are as individual as they are
- **We Develop**
  We plan & provide essential baby & childhood experiences
- **We Protect**
  You can feel assured in knowing our nursery is safe & secure
- **We Listen**
  We welcome and encourage a working partnership between parents and all aston pierpoint staf

- 3 Months - 5 Years
- Monday - Friday 08.00 - 18.00
- Additional hours on request
- Full Time, Part Time & Emergency Days
- House & Gardens designed especially for Children

Please call for a brochure or to arrange a visit.
Tel: **0870 046 3301**, Email: Info@astonpierpoint.com
Please call for Job Vacancy Information

Leading the way in Child Care & Education

nurseries: private & nursery schools (cont.)

Hollygrove Nursery School
The Scout Hall. 020 8941 1022
2^1/$_2$-5yrs

Rectory Day Nursery
Hampton Community College. 020 8941 9854 ext 6

Sunflower Montessori
St Mary's Church Hall. 020 8979 3236
2^1/$_2$-5yrs

Tadpoles Nursery
Carlisle Park Pavillion, Wensleydale Road.
07710 197715
2-5yrs

Tangley Park Day Nursery
10 Tangley Park Road. 020 8979 6866
3mths-5yrs

Hampton Hill
Greenacres Day Nursery School
143b High St. 020 8941 8608
3mths-5yrs

Hampton Hill Nursery School
Greenwood Centre. 020 8287 7113

Ivytree Nursery
United Reform Church. 020 8941 3447
2^1/$_2$-5yrs

Pied Piper Nursery
Staines Rugby Club. 020 8890 7433
2-5yrs

Hanworth
St. George's Day Nursery
St. George's Church Hall. 020 8831 9980
2-5yrs

Haslemere
Asquith Court Nursery
7 College Hill. 01428 645001

Grayswood Nursey School
Grayswood Village Hall. 01428 682936
2^1/$_2$-5yrs

Montessori Nursery School Weyhill
Scout Headquarters. 01428 656840

Timbers Pre-School & Nursery
7 College Hill. 01428 645001
3mths-5yrs

Hinchley Wood
Badgers Nursery
DSS Government Buildings, Hinchley Wood Training Centre. 020 8268 4451
3mths-5yrs

Horley
**CRANBROOK
(THE CHILDRENS HOUSE)**
Crangal Cottage. 01293 823279
2^1/$_2$-5yrs
See advert on page 77

CRANBROOK NURSERY SCHOOL
The Old Post House,
Antlands Lane East. 01293 772561
2-3yrs

CRANBROOK NURSERY SCHOOL
Acorn Cottage, Antlands Lane West
01293 772561
0-2yrs
See advert on page 77

CRANBROOK NURSERY SCHOOL
The Lodge, Antlands Lane East
01293 772561
0-2yrs
See advert on page 77

CRANBROOK NURSERY SCHOOL
Ivy Cottage, Balcombe Road
01293 772561
3-5yrs
See advert on page 77

Kid Co.
Inger Cottage. 01293 775107

Little Jacks
19 Massetts Road. 0129 8382 3500

The Willow Tree Montessori School
80 Lumley Road. 01293 820721
2-4yrs

"Laughter, love and learning"

Our unique nurseries offer quality care and education for all age groups, and a 'funtastic' after school and holiday club for school children

- 24 hour provision -
- flexible attendance options -
- exceptional staff - sensible rates -
- excellent facilities -

Do contact us for further information: Horley

(01293) 772561

The Cranbrook Group

Hounslow

Asquith Court Nurseries
20 Montague Road. 020 8570 4409
1-5yrs

Heston Nursery
c/o David Lloyd leisure. 020 8813 7544

Old Rectory Nursery School
Church Road. 020 8897 3999
18mths-5yrs

St. Paul's Nursery
St. Paul's Hall. 020 8814 1842
2-5yrs

Isleworth

9 Months Nursery
The Grove. 020 8847 0303
www.9monthsnursery.com
12mths-5yrs

De Lacey Montessori School
St. Francis Church Hall. 020 8560 2519
2^1/$_2$-5yrs

Osterley Park Day Nursery
Quaker Meeting House. 020 8847 4042
2-5yrs

Sticky Licky Nursery
13a Worton Road. 020 8569 8163
stickylicky@freenetname.co.uk
3mths-5yrs

West Thames College Nursery
London Road. 020 8326 2318

Kenley

Abbey Wood Grange Day Nursery
16 Church Road. 020 8660 9040

Kew

Barn Nursery School
The Barn Church Hall. 020 8876 6910
2^1/$_2$-5yrs

Please say you saw the ad in
The Local Baby Directory

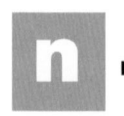

nurseries: private & nursery schools (cont.)

Kew Montessori School
St Lukes House. 020 8940 2791

Monty's Day Nursery
32 Thompson Ave. 020 8392 2336
3mths-5yrs

Kingston-upon-Thames
Albany Park Montessori Nursery School
30 Albany Park Road. 020 8546 9303
3-5yrs

Asquith Court Nursery
49 Kings Road. 020 8974 9773

Asquith Court Nursery
Church Grove. 020 8614 8044

Bushy Park Pre School
Church Grove. 020 8614 8044

Elvira's Montessori Day Nursery
56 Norbiton Avenue. 020 8549 5425

Headstart
71 Richmond Park Road. 020 546 9972
0-5yrs

Kidsenter Nursery
75 Hampden Road. 020 8546 9590
0-5yrs

One, Nine, Seven, Early Years Nursery
197 Richmond Road. 020 8549 9995

Oranges & Lemons Pre-School Nursery
Park Road. 07967 196169
2-5yrs

Park Hill School
8 Queens Road. 020 8546 5496
3-5yrs

Riverside Day Nursery
23 South Lane. 020 8974 8433
0-5yrs

Leatherhead
Greenacres Montessori Nursery School
within Leatherhead Cricket Club
01372 271631

Raleigh Nursery
Northcote Crescent. 01483 281088
2^1/$_2$-5yrs

Long Ditton
Long Ditton Montesorri Children's House
Scout Hall, Betts Way, off Rectory Way
020 8941 6816
2 ^{1}/$_2$-5yrs

Marlborough House Nursery School
Marlborough House. 020 8398 6161
0-5yrs

Mitcham
Cherubs Day Nursery
68 Lewis Road. 020 8646 4644
2-5yrs

Haslemere House Day Nursery
68 Haslemere Avenue. 020 640 0822

Jigsaw Day Nursery
1 Cricket Green. 020 8646 6075
2-5yrs

Nursery on the Green
Mitcham Methodist Church. 020 8648 2446

Spencer Nursery School
Spencer Road. 020 8648 4126
3-5yrs

Morden
Dolphin Day Nursery
St Helier Methodist Church. 020 8288 1945

PETITS ENFANTS DAY NURSERY
2-4 Martin Way. 020 8540 8090
See advert on page 73

PETITS ENFANTS DAY NURSERY
Pheonix College, Central Road
020 8646 7300
3mths-5yrs
See advert on page 73

New Haw
Cherrybrook Nursery
Scotland Bridge Road. 01932 336662

Visit us at
www.babydirectory.com

New Malden
Carousel
Sports Ground. 020 8942 4077

Old Woking
THE ACADEMY PRE-SCHOOL NURSERY
Chris Lane Family Leisure Club, Westfield Avenue. 01483 722113
www.chrislane.com
Quality, private, pre-school educatiion by people that care. Ages 2$^1/_2$-5yrs

Ottershaw
Asquith Court Nursery
Foxhills Country Club. 01932 872050

Cherrywood Nursery
Weybourne House, St Peters. 01932 873303

Toadhall Nursery
The Old School House, Brox Road
01932 874286

Oxted
Swings & Roundabouts
Nursery Way. 01883 722775
6 wks-5yrs

Purley
Bright Sparks Day Nursery
Meadow Hill. 020 8660 2340

Lemon Tree Montessori School
7a Downs Court Road. 020 8668 9826
2$^1/_2$-5yrs

The Purley Day Nursery & Montessori Centre
16 Burcott Road. 020 8645 0105
6mths-5yrs

Purley Nursery School
58 Pampisford Road. 020 8660 5639
3-5yrs

Whytebeams Nursery School
St John The Baptist Parish Centre
020 8660 1641
2$^1/_2$-5yrs

Redhill
Asquith Court Nursery
Bridge House, Royal Earlswood, Princes Road off Brighton Road. 01737 767629

Lilliput Childrens's Centre
West Ave. 01737 789500
4mths-5yrs

Reigate
Asquith Court Nursery
81 Holmesdale Road. 01737 242826

Brantwood Nursery and Baby Unit
6 and 4 Hardwicke Road
01737 242593 and 221622

The Daisy Chain Montessori Nursery
St Lukes Hall. 01737 242001

Leapfrog Day Nurseries
Lesbourne Road. 01737 249109

Richmond
THE CHILDREN'S GARDEN
The Old Chapel, Grove Gardens, off Lower Grove Road. 020 8968 4605
Steiner Kindergarten 3.5-6yrs. Activities: craftwork, baking, French, circle time, organic food. Also run parent/toddler groups

Happy Times Nursery
Grena Road. 020 8334 8720
3mths-5yrs

Ham Nursery School
Ham Day Centre. 020 8332 2445
2$^1/_2$-5yrs

Maria Grey Nursery School
Field House. 020 8940 4350
2$^1/_2$-5yrs. Froebel method

Noahs Ark Nursery
Queens Road. 020 8332 1597
2-5yrs

Windham Nursery School
Windham Road. 020 8940 3765

Runfold
Little Pippins Nursery
9 Tongham Road. 01252 782316

Shepperton
First Steps Nursery
within St Nicholas C of E School. 01932 228841

Springtime Nursery
Rectory Close. 01932 570780

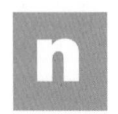

nurseries: private & nursery schools (cont.)

Toad Hall
01932 572525

South Croydon
Beech House School
Church Way. 020 8651 0446

Early Learners
5-8 Blunt Road. 020 8688 0770
6wks-5yrs

Fennies Under 5's Day Nursery
1 St Augustines Avenue. 020 686 5474
4mths-5yrs

Kinderland Day Nursery
1 Normanton Road. 020 8760 0617

Little Learners Day Nursery
Haling Manor High School Grounds
020 8649 7745
3mths-5yrs

Ready Teddy Go
1 Haling Park Road. 020 8667 1669

Staines
KNOWLE GREEN DAY NURSERY (CHILD BASE)
Knowle Green, Staines, TW18 1AJ
01784 464141
knowlegreen@childbase.com
www.childbase.com
We Care As Much As You
See advert on page 71

Little Willows Nursery School
Baptist Church Hall. 01784 461444
2^1/$_2$-5yrs

Roslin's
Rookery Road. 01784 462028

St Peter's Nursery School
Hazelwood House, 38 Richmond Road
01784 455518
2^1/$_2$-5yrs, half day. Rudolth Steiner based

Stoneleigh
Dell Lane Nursery
St John Scout Hut, Dell Lane. 020 8393 0060
2^1/$_2$-5yrs

Time For Tots Ltd
The Old Dairy. 020 8786 8006

Sunbury-on-Thames
Pomfrett Cottage Nursery
37a Thames Street. 01932 779556

Surbiton
ABC Nursery
317 Ewell Road. 020 8399 6498
2-5yrs

Asquith Court Nursery
23 Upper Brighton Road. 020 8390 7744

Buttercups Nursery School
Surbiton Baptist Church. 020 8390 0833
3-5yrs

Childs Play Nursery
31 St Matthews Avenue. 020 8399 7347
3-5yrs

Happy Days Nursery
117 Tolworth Rise North. 020 399 1951
18mths-5yrs

Kidsenter Nursery
St Andrews Hall. 020 8399 0984
0-5yrs

Surbiton Hill Nursery
Alpha Road. 020 8390 2555
3-5yrs

Sutton
Acorn Nursery School
27 Burleigh Road. 020 8641 5038
2^1/$_2$-5yrs

Bubbles Day Nursery For Children
107 Burdon Lane. 020 8642 9318
18mths-5yrs

Buffer Bear Nursery
21B Cheam Road. 020 8643 5278

Elmbrook Christian Nursery
Elmbrook Chapel. 020 8641 7326
3-5yrs

Visit us at
www.babydirectory.com

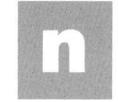

Hopscotch Day Nursery
16 Avenue Road. 020 773 8142

PETITS ENFANTS DAY NURSERY
BLUE FIRS
128 Grove Road. 020 8661 2201
18mths-5yrs
See advert on page 73

TEDDIES
14 Sherwood Park Road. 020 8770 0261
3mths-5yrs

Thomas Wall Nursery School
Robin Hood Lane. 020 8642 5666
3-5yrs

Tadworth
Buffer Bear Nursery
Tadworth Court. 01737 351907

The Lanes Kindergarten
Breech Lane. 01737 814207
2¹/₂-5yrs

St Johns Nursery School
59 The Avenue. 01737 813032
2¹/₂-5yrs

Teddington
Asquith Court Nursery
16 Cedar Road. 020 8943 4330

Holly House Nursery
7 Stanley Road. 020 8943 9901
2mths-5yrs

Little Munster's
24 Munster Road. 020 8977 5068
2-5yrs

PETITS ENFANTS DAY NURSERY
81 Fulwell Road. 020 8943 2227
3mths-5yrs
See advert on page 73

PETITS ENFANTS DAY NURSERY
52 Church Road. 020 8977 0202
3mths-5yrs
See advert on page 73

Thames Ditton
Elvira's Montessori Day Care Ltd
1 Weston Avenue. 020 8398 1497
2-5yrs

Brook House Nursery
110 Cole Park Road, Twickenham

24-place Nursery caring for
children aged 5 months to five years.
Friendly, family home, qualified staff,
OFSTED-approved.

Laura Hookway RGN

020 8892 4853

PETITS ENFANTS DAY NURSERY
1-2 Mercer Close. 020 8398 9491
3mths-5yrs
See advert on page 73

Thornton Heath
Allens Montessori Day Nursery
47 Beulah Road. 020 8771 2728

Bonny Belles Kindergarten Day Nursery
19 Liverpool Road. 020 8768 0494

Buffer Bear Nursery
Woodcote Ward, Mayday Hospital
020 8401 3819

Croydon Montessori School
37 County Road. 020 8240 0076
2-5yrs

King Fishers Day Nursery
89 Brigstock Road. 020 8665 5429
2-5yrs

Little Angels Day Nursery
57 Richmond Road. 020 8684 0338

Tolworth
Chatterbox Day Nursery
The Studios. 020 399 9429
2-5yrs

PETITS ENFANTS DAY NURSERY
Tolworth Hospital. 020 8339 9800
See advert on page 73

Twickenham
BROOK HOUSE NURSERY
110 Cole Park Road. 020 8892 4853
5mths-5yrs

nurseries: private & nursery schools (cont.)

Buttercup Nursery
Isleworth Explorers Club. 020 8560 4539
18mths-5yrs

Crane Park Nursery
270 Staines Road. 020 8894 0116
3mths-5yrs

Jane's Montessori
13 Rosslyn Road. 020 8891 2752
2^1/$_2$-5yrs

Lebanon Park Day Nursery
Little Ferry Road. 020 8607 9987
2-5yrs

Merrygold Montessori School
Kneller Road. 020 8898 0962

Montessori Cellars Nursery School
219 Richmond Road. 020 8892 2620

Peaches Nursery
Erncroft Way. 020 8580 9402
2^1/$_2$-5yrs

Pinocchio Nursery School
All Saints Church Hall. 020 8891 3195

Sunflower Montessori School
8 Victoria Road. 020 8891 2675
2^1/$_2$-7yrs

TEDDIES NURSERIES
57 Holly Road. 020 8744 1531
See advert on page 69

TEDDIES NURSERIES
3 March Road. 020 8744 9643
See advert on page 69

Tic Toc Nursery School
298-300 Staines Road. 020 8898 4079
3mths-5yrs

Twickenham Park Day Nursery
Cambridge Road. 020 8892 0872
3mths-5yrs

Windsor Kindergarten
St. Mary's Church Hall. 020 8892 3651
2^1/$_2$-5yrs

Virginia Water
Trotsworth Nursery School
rear of Virginia Water Library. 01344 843289
2^1/$_2$-5yrs

Windsor Montessori School
Cramond. 01344 844592

Wallington
Jackanory Nursery
21 Hawthorn Road. 020 8669 2988
18mths-5yrs

JANCETT DAY NURSERY
55 Ross Road. 020 8773 8142
See advert on page 67

Kindergarten Nursery School
18 Mollison Drive. 020 8647 2811

Lindbergh Play Centre
Lindbergh Road. 020 8669 6658
0-5yrs, Mother toddler group, Mon, Tues, Thurs, Fri

Startel Nursery
Holmwood Gardens. 020 8669 4898

Wordsworth Pre-School Nursery
4 Wordsworth Road. 020 8669 6876

Walton-on-Thames
Child Development & Enrichment Centre
Felcott Road. 01932 252858
3mths-8yrs

Child's Play Baby Centres
Manor Road. 01932 226975
3mths -5yrs

Lilliput Childrens Centre
Burwood Road. 01932 252202
4mths-5yrs

Stagecoach Montessori School
The Courthouse, Elm Grove. 01932 253528
2-5yrs

Visit us at
www.babydirectory.com

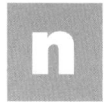

Village Nursery School
Octagon Road. 01932 230611

Warlingham
Whytebeam Nursery School
rear of 192 Limpsfield Road. 01883 625149
2-5yrs

West Byfleet
Discovery Montessori School
within West Byfleets Infants School
01932 354284

West Dorking
Asquith Court Nursery
The White House, Dorking Hospital
01306 742143

West Ewell
Emmanuel Nursery School
St Francis Church Hall, Ruxley Lane
01428 722787
3-5yrs

Little Saints Pre-School
All Saints Community Hall, Fulford Road
020 8393 1777
2^1/$_2$-5yrs

Ruxley Methodist Church Nursery
Ruxley Methodist Church Hall, Ruxley Lane.
020 8397 6212
2^1/$_2$-5yrs

Weybridge
Brooklands Healthtrack Creche
Brooklands Road. 01932 858560
3mths-5yrs, membership only

Cherrylands Nursery
Sopwith Drive. 01932 354175

Whitton
Murray Park Nursery
Whitton Baptist Church, Hounslow Road
020 8894 9947
30mths-5yrs

Squirrels Day Nursery
Nelson Road. 020 8893 3465

Whitton Day Nursery
Willowdene Close. 020 8893 3073
2-5yrs

Whyteleafe
ABC Day Nursery
Whyteleafe Hill. 01883 627211
3mths-5yrs

Cruwys Cherubs Nursery School
St Thomas of Canterbury Hall. 01883 626983
2^1/$_2$-5yrs

Windlesham
Hatton Hill Day Nursery
Hatton Hill. 01276 474764

Woking
Christopher Robin Day Nurseries
31 Claremont Avenue. 01483 757507

Kiddiwinks Child Care Ltd
Bishop David Brown School. 01932 350039
3mths-5yrs

Leapfrog Day Nurseries
50 Cavell Way. 01483 797966

Murrell's Playschool
28 Abbey Road. 01483 725148
2^1/$_2$-5yrs

Noah's Ark Day Nursery
Blackhorse Road. 01483 233832

Peter Pan Pre-School Nursery
St. Thomas Church. 01483 799838
2^1/$_2$-5yrs

Ripley Day Nursery
Ripley C of E School. 01483 222020

TEDDIES NURSERIES
15 The Grove. 01372 210904
See advert on page 69

Woldingham
Woldingham Nursery Class
Village Hall. 01883 380804
Mornings 9.15am-12noon. 2^1/$_2$-5yrs

Worcester Park
Buzy Bees Day Nursery
Longfellow Road. 020 8335 3537

Worcester Park Montessori Nursery
Wesley Hall. 020 8330 6630
2^1/$_2$-5yrs

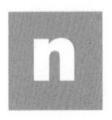

nursery furniture & decor

(see also murals, nursery goods)

LIONWITCHWARDROBE
020 8265 8449
info@lionwitchwardrobe.co.uk
www.lionwitchwardrobe.co.uk
Hand-crafted contemporary oak furniture and accessories for style-conscious parents

Ragazzi Nursery Furniture
c/o The Vending Corporation, Avenue 1, Station Lane, Witney, Oxfordshire
01993 774601
www.ragazzi.com

The Children's Furniture Company
PO Box 31681 London SW2 5ZE
020 7737 7303
www.thechildrensfurniturecompany.com
Exclusive range of children's furniture in hardwoods or painted finishes

nursery goods

(see also clothing shops, nearly new, mail order, murals & painted furniture, nearly new, nursery furniture & decor)

BABY BLISS
020 8568 4913
Feeding pillows, nappy buckets, maternity bras etc

Babysfirstwave
810 771 1828
www.babysfirstwave.com
The first drive home car flag

Little Stars
020 8621 4378/020 8537 0980
www.littlestars.co.uk
Buy or hire your new baby equipment today

Ashford
Rose Prams
17 Feltham Road. 01784 256664

Ashtead
The Children's Room
102 The Street. 01372 273436

Camberley
BabyGear
1 Portesbery Road. 01276 20404

Chessington
Nippers
The Waffrons. 020 8398 3114

Cobham
Little B's The Baby Shop
7 Holly Parade. 01932 868294

Coulsdon
Kid Equip
187 Chipstead Valley Road. 01737 552545

Croydon
Allders
020 8256 7000

Baby Nest
230 London Road. 020 8667 9363

Cuddles Baby Shop
109 South End. 020 8649 7782

Dorking
Baby Room
2 St. Martin's Walk. 01306 887575

Epsom
Kids Gear
29 Waterloo Road. 01372 721450

Feltham
Happicraft Ltd
144 The Centre. 020 8890 4211

Trading Places
112 The Centre. 020 8893 2960

Guildford
The Baby's Room
11 Tunsgate. 01483 578984

London SW3
NURSERY WINDOW
83 Walton Street. 020 7581 3358
www.nurserywindow.co.uk
Exclusive accessories, fabrics, wallpapers, bedding and furniture

Please say you saw the ad in
The Local Baby Directory

Southampton
BABYNEEDS SUPERSTORE
491-497 Bitterne Road East. 02380 454544
info@baby-needs.co.uk
www.baby-needs.co.uk
Massive range of prams, buggies, cots, furniture, bedding, car seats, toys etc

Surbiton
Mothers Nest
25 The Broadway. 020 8390 6581

Thornton Heath
Mac's Best For Less Babyware
37 High Street. 020 8683 3682

Twickenham
Happicraft Ltd
46-48 London Road. 020 8892 5262

JAC & BETY
14 Church Street
020 8892 3776
Unique & practical products for babies & children

The Nursery Window

exclusive accessories, fabrics, wallpapers, bedding and furniture providing you with the total package for your childs bedroom from birth upwards

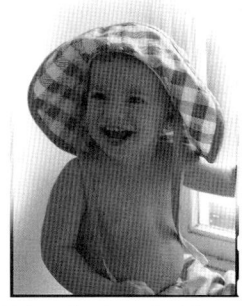

Available by mail order or direct from our shop

Telephone 020 7581 3358
www.nurserywindow.co.uk
83 WALTON STREET LONDON   SW3 2HP

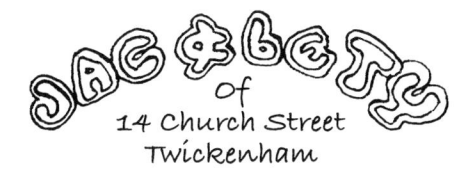

JAC & BETY
of
14 Church Street
Twickenham

Aromatherapy
Bambino Mio
Bonne Nuit
Collins & Hall
Daisy Roots, Hippychick
Flap Happy
FNUC
Handmade Toys
Kent & Carey

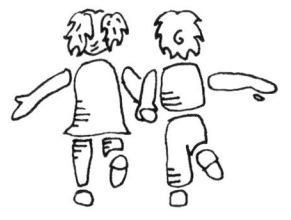

Unique & practical products for babies & children aged 2-3yrs

Kooshies
New Potatoes
North American Bear
Osh Kosh
Sleepi Cot
Sposh UV Sunwear
Spottiswood
The Nursery Company
Tripp Trapp Chair

Tel: 020 8892 3776

nutrition

www.zitawest.com
0870 668899

British Dietetic Association
0121 200 8080

Foresight: Association for Preconceptual Care
01483 427839

Wellbeing Eating for Pregnancy Helpline
0114 242 4084

Guildford
Tim Foulsham
Vale End Chinese Health Clinic. 01483 202556

London
Centre for Nutritional Medicine
114 Harley Street. 020 7224 5053

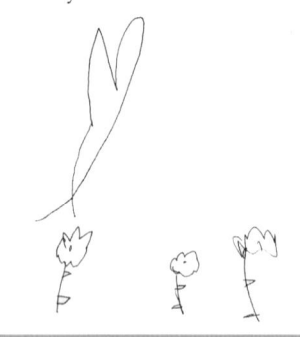

organic

(see also health food shops, food, nappies: cloth & other)

Soil Association
0117 929 0661
info@soilassociation.org
www.soilassociation.org
Loads of information about everything organic!

Abel & Cole
020 7737 3648
www.abel-cole.co.uk
Home delivery box scheme

Green People Co. Ltd
01444 401444
Skincare

Lavender Blue
0118 969 3148
Organic skincare for mother & baby

Open Eye
020 8286 4324
Home delivery of organic produce in Twickenham, Hampton, Isleworth and Teddington.

Simply Organic
020 7622 5006
Home delivery

Guildford
Surrey Organics
01483 300424
Box scheme

Morden
Greenshoot
22a Crown Lane. 01483 203179

Redhill
Greener Greens Box Delivery
Nutfield Road. 01737 766792

Reigate
Octavia's Organics
7 Princes Lane, Woodhatch. 01737 244155

Richmond
Organic World
23 Friars Stile Road. 020 8940 0414
Organic meat and dried goods

Twickenham
Gaia Wholefoods
123 St Margarets Road. 020 8892 2262

osteopaths

(see also craniosacral therapy)

Cranial osteopathy can be particularly beneficial to babies and children. It is often recommended following a difficult birth or in treating conditions such as glue ear.

General Osteopathic Council
Osteopathy House, 176 Tower Bridge Road, London, SE1. 020 7357 6655

Addlestone
Addlestone Therapy Centre
164 Station Road. 01932 831616

Ashford
Ashford Osteopathic Clinic
23 Feltham Road. 01784 255535
Also cranial osteopathy

Chessington
The Osteopathic Centre
9a Mansfield Road. 020 8397 8629

East Molesey
Hampton Court Health Clinic
Cardinal House, 7 Wolsey Road. 020 8481 7606
Also cranial osteopathy

MARTINE L. FAURE-ALDERSON
HEALTH CLINIC
187 Ember Lane. 020 8398 6943
Also cranial osteopathy

Epsom
Morag Christie
16 Denham Road. 01372 803604

Farnham
Saffron Ray
Oak Park Osteopathic Clinic, Heath Lane, Crondall. 01252 672265
saffronray@gu139ny.freeserve.co.uk

Kingston-upon-Thames
Kingston Osteopaths
145a London Road. 020 8546 5995

London
Osteopathic Centre for Children
109 Harley Street. 020 7486 6160

Teddington
Janet Bell
Teddington Memorial Hospital,
Hampton Road. 020 8408 8213

Twickenham
Oak Lane Osteopaths
Oak Lane Medical Centre, 6 Oak Lane
020 8891 3400

SAMANTHA HURST, B.SC. (OST)
REGISTERED OSTEOPATH
20 The Green. 020 8893 3084

Samantha Hurst B.Sc.(Ost)
Registered Osteopath

Pregnancy is responsible for significant changes in posture and in many cases this gives rise to back pain and discomfort.

Many women find relief from gentle osteopathic treatment both before and after birth.

Treatment of you and your children available in a child – friendly clinic.

Tel: 07050 186648,
020 8893 3084
for further details

20 The Green, Twickenham

THE MARIS PRACTICE
13 Baylis Mews, Amyand Park Road
020 8891 3400
themarispractice@hotmail.com
www.stellamaris.org
A group of osteopaths all experienced in the treatment of children.

Wiltshire
THE SUTHERLAND SOCIETY
15a Church Street, Bradford on Avon, Wiltshire. 0845 6030680
www.cranial.org.uk
For information regarding the cranial approach, including the treatmrnt of babies & children

Please say you saw the ad in
The Local Baby Directory

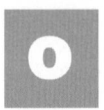

outings

(see also country parks, farms, indoor adventure playcentres, museums, parks, theatres, theme parks, zoos)

Always ring to check opening times and avoid disappointment. If you are travelling outside the area covered by this Baby Directory, don't forget to arm yourself with the necessary Local Baby Directory. We now cover

- Bristol, Bath & Somerset
- Herts & Middlesex
- London
- Oxfordshire, Bucks & Berks
- South Wales
- Sussex & Hampshire

Alton Towers
Alton. 0870 520 4060
Jct 15 off M6

Bekonscot Model Village
Warwick Road, Beaconsfield. 01494 672919

Changing the Guard
Buckingham Palace, The Mall.
Daily 11.30am from April to end of July.
Alternate days in winter.

Chessington World of Adventures
Leatherhead Road, Chessington. 01372 729 560
Theme park and zoo. Jct 9 off M25 or A3

Chiltern Open Air Museum
Newlands Park, Calfton Lane, Gorelands.
01494 871117
Closed in winter

GODSTONE FARM
Tilburstow Hill Road, Godstone
01883 742546
www.godstonefarm.co.uk
See advert on page 24

Great Cockrow Miniature Railway
Hardwick Lane, Near Chertsey. 01932 255514
Sundays in the summer.

Hampton Court Palace
East Molesey. 020 8781 9500
Good tea rooms. Children's trail and maze.
M25 Jct 10, A307 or Jct 12, A308.

Heathrow Airport Visitor Centre
Newell Road, off the Northern Perimeter, Heathrow Airport. 020 8745 6655

HMS Belfast
Morgan's Lane, off Tooley Street
020 7940 6300

HORTON PARK CHILDREN'S FARM
Horton Lane, Epsom. 01372 743984
www.hortonpark.co.uk
See adverts on page 24 & 89

Imax Cinema
Roundabout, Waterloo Station. 020 7902 1234
UK's biggest screen

Legoland
Winkfield Road, Windsor. 0990 040 404
Jct 6 off M4, Jct 3 off M3. Train from Waterloo + shuttle bus.

London Aquarium
County Hall, Westminster Bridge Road
020 7967 8000

London Frog Tours
County Hall, Riverside Buildings, Westminster Bridge Road. 020 7928 3132
Amphibious craft, river and road tour Summer only

The London Butterfly House
Syon Park, Brentford. 020 8560 0378
Tropical butterflies, toads, iguanas. Aquarium. Can be combined with Snakes and Ladders indoor adventure playground and the garden centre

The London Eye
Jubilee Gardens. 0870 5000 600
Bit dull for tinies – and no getting off half-way!

London Planetarium
Marylebone Road. 020 7935 6861

Look Out Discovery Park
Nine Mile Road, Bracknell. 01344 868 222
Environmental family park. Combine with Coral Reef. M4, Jct 10, A322 signs for Bagshot

Please say you saw the ad in
The Local Baby Directory

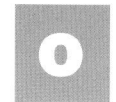

Lockwood Donkey Sanctuay
Home for retired donkeys
(Plus Horses, sheep, goats, lamas)

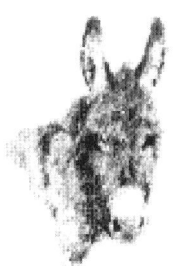

In the Guinness book of records for the 'worlds oldest donkey'

Farm Cottage, Sanhills, Wormley, Surrey GU8 5UX
01428 682 409
Open 9-5, 7 days a week, 365 days a year

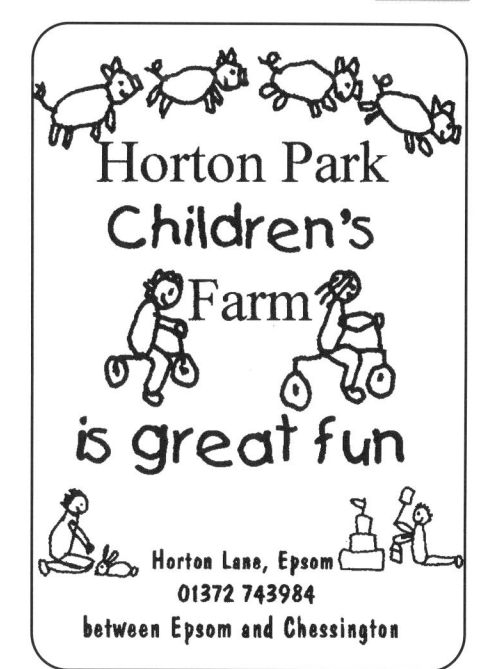

Horton Park Children's Farm is great fun

Horton Lane, Epsom
01372 743984
between Epsom and Chessington

LOCKWOOD DONKEY SANCTUARY
Farm Cottage, Sanhills. 01428 682409

Madame Tussaud's
Baker Street. 0870 400 3000
Too frightening for tinies. And the queue…
Tube to Baker Street

Osterley Park House
01494 755566
National Trust property, large grounds, tearoom, house not suitable for pushchairs or backpacks

Royal Mews
Buckingham Palace. 020 7930 4832

Thames Ditton Miniature Railway
Claygate Lane. 020 8398 3985
1st Sunday of the month, Easter-October

Thorpe Park
Staines Road, Chertsey. 01932 569393
White knuckle water rides

Tower of London
Tower Hill. 020 7709 0765
Mon-Sat 9-6pm, winter 9.30-5pm. Sun 10-6pm, winter 10-5pm. Tube to Tower Hill

Walter Rothschild Zoological Museum
Akeman Street, Tring. 01442 824181
Victorian animals

Windsor Castle
01753 868286

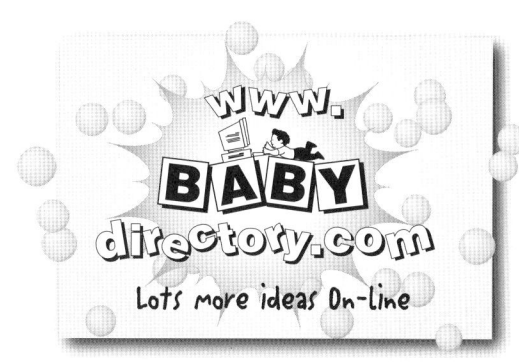

www.babydirectory.com
Lots more ideas On-line

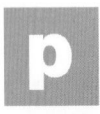

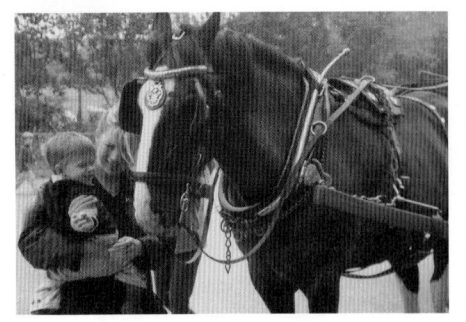

parent & toddler groups

(see also playgroups)

These are mainly for parents or carers with children under three years, but some extend to under 5s. Usually run by parents, they are held in church halls, etc, and carers remain with the children. There is usually a small charge. Ring your local council *(see councils)* for venues near you, or check notice boards in clinics, hospitals and libraries

parentcraft classes & advice

Centre for Parenting Studies
Merton College. 020 8640 3001

Crechendo Training
020 8772 8160
www.crechendo.com
Will run courses for groups in your home

Parentalk
020 7450 9073

Parenting Education & Support Forum
020 7284 8370

parks & playgrounds

(see also adventure playgrounds, outings)

Brentford
Boston Manor Park
Boston Manor Road. 020 8560 5441
Playground cunningly situated virtually under the motorway. Nature trail, pond, scarey woodlands and copious dog mess. Annual Civil War battle re-enactments

Syon Park
Brentford. 020 8560 0883
Lake, train in summer. Entry charge
See also outings, indoor adventure playground

Cobham
Painshill Park Trust
Portsmouth Road. 01932 868113

Farnham
Forest Enterprise
Bucks Horn Oak. 01420 23666

Hampton Court
Bushy Park
Huge sandpit, model boats, café, deer

Hanscombe
Winkworth Arboretum
01483 208477

Isleworth
Osterley Park
Jersey Road. 020 8232 5050
Extensive grounds of large house. Good teas in old stables. Lake, gardens and large "wild" green areas. Cows and horses in surrounding fields. Great bluebells (worth coming from afar)

Kew
Kew Royal Botanic Gardens
020 8940 1171
Worth the price of entry even in bleak midwinter to gain entrance to palm houses. Good cafes, wonderful aquarium (down a buggy unfriendly spiral stair in the Palm House). No balls or dogs

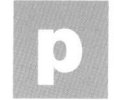

London
Chiswick House
Burlington Lane. 020 8995 0508
Great woodland with hidden pathways, excellent child-friendly café with lawn for games in front (w/e only in winter).

Dukes Meadow
Off Great Chertsey Road, behind Chiswick New Pool.
Secret and empty playground. Good climbing structure and swings, and unusual elastic climbing frame to have a boing on. Beware broken glass

Ravenscourt Park
020 8741 2051
Three areas for children. Good swings, slides, balancing equipment. Under 5's centre. Unusual wooden structures. Dog-free zones. Excellent paddling pool. Sandpit. Slow café

Lightwater
Lightwater Country Park
The Avenue. 01276 479582
Also small leisure centre

Richmond
Richmond Park
020 8948 3209
Largest royal park in London. Wide open spaces, trees, lots of deer, lakes, horses etc. Also the Isabella Plantation, an enclosed area, beautiful especially in spring

Twickenham
Crane Park
Nature reserve. Good bike path along River Crane

Marble Hill Park
Richmond Road. 020 8892 5115
Adventure playground, Under 5's centre, café (Mar-Oct)

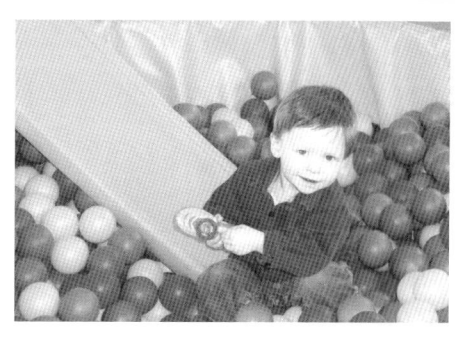

party entertainers

Adam Ant
020 8959 1045

Albert and Friends
020 8237 1170
Teach circus skills 15mths upwards

BLUEBERRY PLAYSONGS PARTIES!
020 8677 6871
blueberry@clara.co.uk
See advert under music

Bumble The Clown
020 8399 6007

Cookie Crumbles
0845 601 4173
carola@cookiecrumbles.net
5-16yrs

Crêchendo Children's Parties
020 8772 8140
events@crechendo.com
www.crechendo.com
1-2yrs

Fun Food Academy
01243 573975
Children's cookery birthday parties

Graham Lee's Magic
020 8644 1983

The Great Custardo
020 8542 9397
www.custardo.co.uk
Circus workshops

TWIZZLE
PARTIES & EVENTS

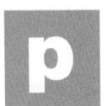

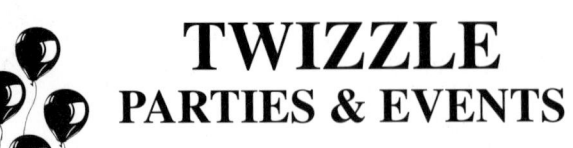

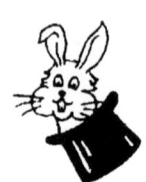

We provide the best in children's party fun and entertainment

Recommended by The Observer & Tatler

- Magic, games, prizes, balloon modelling and puppet shows for all ages
- Discos • Bouncy castles
- Fabulous theme parties
- Table and chair hire, food and party bags also available

We offer a complete party service!

Tel: 020 8392 6788

---

party entertainers (cont.)

HOUSE PARTY
08707 657575
contact@my-houseparty.com
www.my-houseparty.com
We do all the work- you have all the fun!

Jolly Dolly's Magic
01932 786023

Jumpin' Jacks
07866 341779
www.jumpinjacks.co.uk

Kids Works
020 8755 1583
Games & football parties

LITTLE BLISTERS
2 South Lodge, Ham Common
020 8948 3874
Wonderful children's parties: Flossie the Fairy, Sealily the Mermaid or Kitty Willow

Loopy Lou's Puppet show
01932 245590

Mr Mysto
0800 0188118

Michelle Smith
020 8287 6870
michelle@kidspartytime.biz
Party organiser

TWIZZLE ENTERTAINMENT
020 8392 6788
The best children's party fun and entertainment

Walligog the Wizard
0118 9730737

Visit us at
www.babydirectory.com

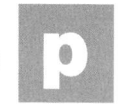

LITTLE BLISTERS
PARTY ENTERTAINERS
With FLOSSIE THE FAIRY
PEARL THE MERMAID
THE MAGICAL PUSSYCAT
Magical shows, face painting,
Music, balloons, games...
Tel: 020 8948 3874

BOUNCE AWAY
For Hire

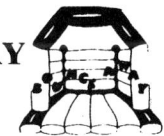

Choice of bouncy castles
Children's tables & chairs

SW London 020 8788 2647

party equipment

(see also fancy dress, party entertainers)

mail order

Abacus Entertainment
020 8777 9611

Adam Ants Partyware
020 8959 1045

Ball Bounce
020 8977 2627

BOUNCE AWAY
020 8788 2647
Bouncy castles, tables, chairs for hire

I love balloons ltd
020 8904 0004
www.Iloveballoons.co.uk
Children's themed party balloons, party décor, table centrepieces and party accessories

Minimarkee
020 8741 2777

Party zone
01277 226999
www.partyzone.co.uk
Themed children's party tableware/loot bags/meal boxes & party toys

Partyco
020 8995 1782
www.partyco.co.uk

Party Pieces
01635 201844

Partyworks
0870 2402103
www.partybypost.co.uk

retail

Banstead
D & M Transformation
33 Partridge Mead. 01737 352373
Balloon decorator

Caterham
Party Stop
24 Croydon Road. 01883 331333

Chessington
Bit of a Do
Unit 4, Chessington North Station,
Bridge Road. 020 8391 5466

Cobham
Non Stop Party Shop Ltd
35 High Street. 01932 868675

East Molesey
Balloon Creations Ltd
3 Palace Gate House, Hampton Court
020 8399 5001

Balloonatics
90 Stoneleigh Park Road. 020 8393 7499

Epsom
Masquerade
360 Kingston Road, Ewell. 020 8393 2626

Please say you saw the ad in
The Local Baby Directory

party equipment (cont.)

Guildford
The Party Shop
6 Milkhouse Gate. 01483 576262

Haslemere
Hokey Cokey
23a Liphook Road, Shottermill. 01428 644179

Kew
The Balloon Works
233 Sandycombe Road. 020 8948 8157

Party Pieces
020 8876 6163

Kingston-upon-Thames
123 Partee
The Coach House, Barge Walk. 020 8614 5620

Euphoria
112 Barnfield Avenue. 020 8549 1947

Leatherhead
Up & Away Balloons of Leatherhead
Firwood House, 12 Lower Road, Fetcham
01372 375255

Lingfield
High Flyers
New Cottage Farm, Crowhurst Lane
01342 892554
Balloons & gifts

Richmond
The Party House
6 Duke Street. 020 8332 6610

Sutton
Party Superstore
43 Times Square, High Street. 020 8661 7323

Teddington
The Fun Factory
14 The Causeway. 020 8977 1006

Walton-on-Thames
Bissons Blooms & Balloons
29 Church Street. 01932 244600

West Horsley
Abacus Baby & Partyhire
01483 285142
Tables, chairs, bouncy castles etc

Weybridge
Non-Stop Party Shop Ltd
4 Church Street. 01932 845319

Worcester Park
A Present World of Balloons & Decorations
6 Elmstead Gardens. 020 8335 3530

party venues

Try swimming pools, indoor adventure playgrounds, church halls, arts centres, ceramic cafes and leisure centres

Brentford
Brentford Fountain Leisure Centre
658 Chiswick High Road. 020 8994 9596

Kingston-upon-Thames
World Of Children Playcare Centre
Bentalls Centre. 020 8974 8502
1-8yrs

Old Woking
KIDSPORTS
Chris Lane Family Leisure Club,
Westfield Avenue. 01483 722113
www.chrislane.com
Fun, unusual, quality venues for ages 2-10yrs, themed

Richmond
Lollipop Club
Old Deer Park. 020 8332 7436
Term time only. 0-5yrs

Sutton
VILLAGE CERAMICS
31 Station Way, Cheam Village
020 8661 7837
charlotte@villageceramics.co.uk
www.villageceramics.co.uk
See advert under ceramics

Visit us at
www.babydirectory.com

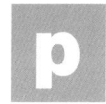

paternity testing

CELLMARK DIAGNOSTICS
PO Box 265, Abingdon, Oxfordshire
01235 528000
www.cellmark.co.uk
5-day DNA test. Phone customer services for confidential advice

personal trainers

(see exercise classes, health clubs with crèches)

London Academy of Personal Fitness
0870 4423231
www.lapf.co.uk

Estelle Pendleton
020 8255 4592

Lysta Perry
020 8994 8118
Ante and post natal personal fitness training

photographers specialising in babies & children

Farzi Bantin
020 8891 3059
photography@farzibantin.com

SOPHIE CARR
07957 218864

Vibeke Dahl
020 8876 8113

Jo-Jo's Children's Photography
020 8995 3257

Laurence Photography
01372 722522

Little Shots of Horrors
020 8546 5182

Ken Nemar Photography

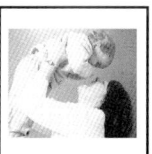

Special Offer
To Baby Directory Readers

Capture The Magic Of Your Little Treasures With A Professional Studio Portrait Session

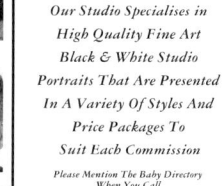

For Only £19.95
(Normal Studio Fee £60)

Our Studio Specialises in High Quality Fine Art Black & White Studio Portraits That Are Presented In A Variety Of Styles And Price Packages To Suit Each Commission

Please Mention The Baby Directory When You Call

Creating Beautiful Pictures For You To Treasure

020 8398 3081 (Esher)
Ken Nemar Photography
FREEPOST SEA 12682 Esher KT10 8BR

KEN NEMAR
52 The Woodlands, Esher. 020 8398 3081
kgnemar@aol.com

David Stubbs Photography
020 8898 4178

physiotherapists

The Chartered Society of Physiotherapists
14 Bedford Row. 020 7306 6666
Contact for details of qualified physios in your area

Richmond
Richmond Physiotherapy
16 King Street. 020 8332 1132

Please say you saw the ad in
The Local Baby Directory

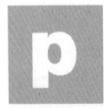

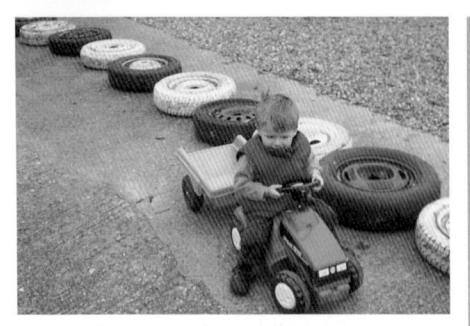

playgroups

Below are listed a few of the many hundreds of playgroups in the area. They are usually on for one or two sessions per week and children need to be accompanied. Contact the Pre-School Learning Alliance on 020 7833 0991 for up-to-date information on your local playgroup. For non PLA playgroups, contact the Under 8s section at your local council (see councils).

PRE-SCHOOL LEARNING ALLIANCE
National Centre, 69 Kings Cross Road, London, WC1. 020 7833 0991
www.pre-school.org.uk
Leading early years provider with 16,000 pre-schools and 20,000 adults on their training courses each year

Bookham
Say & Play Pre-School Group
Edenside Clinic, 33 Edenside Road
01372 450472
Speech & Language therapy facility

Cheam
St Paul's Playgroup
St Paul's Church Centre, Howell Hill
020 8224 9838
2-5yrs

Cobham
Playtime
Scout Hut, Hogshill Lane. 01483 285 284
Sessions in Cobham, Fetcham and Effingham for 2-3yrs

Epsom
Blenheim Playgroup
01372 743196
3-5yrs

Epsom Downs Playgroup
Village Hall, Rosebury Road, Langley Vale
01372 271788
2-5yrs

Ewell
Little Ferns Playgroup
The Scout Hut, 106 West Street. 0589 548350
2¹/₂-5yrs

Godalming
Orchard Community Playgroup
17a Elmside, Milford. 01483 427493
2¹/₂-5yrs

Guildford
Bramley Pre-Schools Group
Bramley Village Hall, Hall Road, Bramley
01483 894016

Bright Star Playgroup
United Reformed Church Hall,
83 Portsmouth Road. 01483 565298
2¹/₂-5yrs

Haslemere
Camelsdale Playgroup
Church Hall, School Road. 01428 643495
2¹/₂-5yrs

Kingston-upon-Thames
Play People Playgroup
Canbury Park Church, Park Road
020 8974 8938

Leatherwood
Playaway Pre-School
within Fetcham Infant School, School Lane, Fetcham. 01372 361130

Reigate
Reigate Parish School Playgroup
Reigate Parish Church School,
91 Blackborough Road. 01737 225649

St Margarets
Munchkins
All Souls' Church Hall, Northcote Road

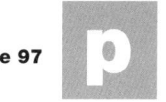

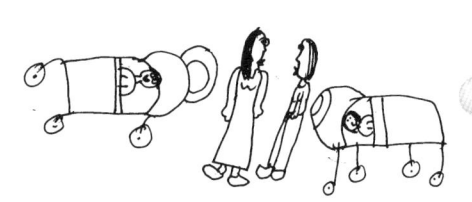

Stoneleigh
Crescent Playgroup
Stoneleigh Methodist Church Hall,
Stoneleigh Crescent. 020 8393 9743
2-5yrs

Sparrows Pre-School Playgroup
Stoneleigh Adult Education, Waverley Road
020 8873 1453
2^1/$_2$-5yrs

Sutton
Caterpillar Pre-school
Thomas Wall Centre, Benhill Avenue
020 8715 7735

Thames Ditton
Play Away
Thames Ditton Infant School. 020 8224 5132
2-3yrs

Twickenham
St James's Playgroup
St James's Church Hall, Radnor Road
020 8894 7419
Friday mornings

Walton-on-Thames
Burwood Playgroup
Burhill Infant School, Pleasant Place, Hersham
01932 240026
2^1/$_2$-5yrs

Woking
Woodlands Pre-School Group
within Barnsbury County Infant School,
Hawthorn Road. 01483 772322

Worcester Park
Auriol Park Playgroup
Salisbury Road. 020 8393 0643
2-5yrs

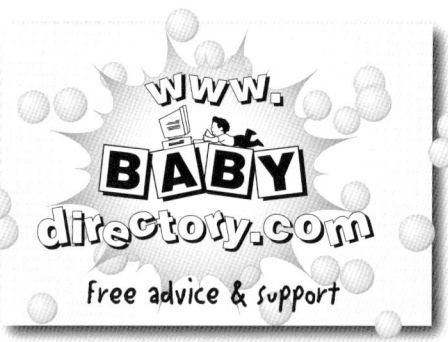

postnatal support & information

(see also breastfeeding, helplines: postnatal advice)

National Childbirth Trust
Alexandra House, Oldham Terrace,
London, W3. 0870 444 8707
Ask for your local branch contact or postnatal co-ordinator

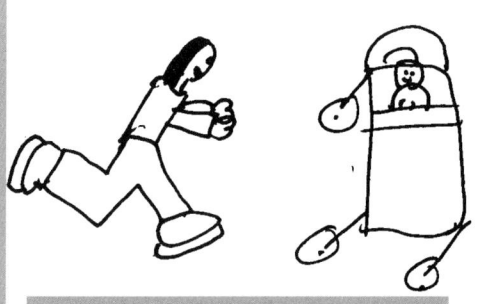

pram & buggy repair

For details of major manufacturers ask at the shop where you bought the pram, or check our list of manufacturers and suppliers

Barnes Buggy Repair Centre
278 Upper Richmond Road, London, SW15
020 8543 0505

Cottam Baby Carriage's
3 Bramcote Parade, Cricket Green, Mitcham
020 8648 4397

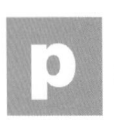

LIFE offers a care and counselling service committed to the unborn and to anyone facing difficulties arising from pregnancy or from the effects of abortion.
Free pregnancy testing, pregnancy counselling, practical support and help with accommodation where needed.
Please contact LIFE Pregnancy on

**Helpline
01483 579773 or
020 8397 6199**
(Please check for Centre opening hours)

**National Helpline
01926 311511**
9.00am to 9.00pm daily

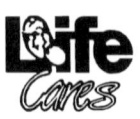

pregnancy testing

Guildford
LIFE PREGNANCY CARE CENTRE
01483 579773
www.guildfordlife.org.uk

Kingston-upon-Thames
LIFE PREGNANCY CARE CENTRE
020 8397 6199

W.Croydon
LIFE Pregnancy Care Centre
57a London Road. 020 8688 1985
10-1.30pm Mon-Fri, 10-12pm Sat

premature babies

Bliss: National Charity for the New Born
68 South Lambeth Road, London, SW8
0500 618140

www.premature-babies.co.uk

psychologists & psychotherapists

Association of Child Psychotherapists
020 8458 1609

Child Psychotherapy Trust
Star House, 104-108 Grafton Road, London, NW5. 020 7284 1355

Child Consultants
27a Harley Place, London, W1. 020 7637 3177

LKA Consultants
01883 626161
Psychology assessments

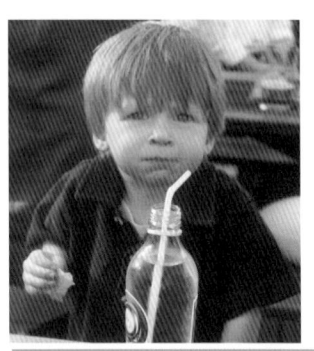

pubs with gardens or playrooms

Croydon
Hare & Hounds
325 Purley Way. 020 8688 0420

Dorking
Dukes Head Hotel
Beare Green. 01306 711778

Elstead
The Woolpack
The Green. 01252 703106
Family room and playground

Hampton Hill
The Windmill
Windmill Road

Mortlake
The Ship Tavern
Ship Lane, off Richmond Road. 020 8876 1439

Richmond
The Marlborough
46 Friar Stile Road. 020 8940 0572

Teddington
Anchor
Playground. Nice location next to Teddington Lock

Twickenham
Prince Blucher
Staines Road

Weybridge
Victoria
Woodham Lane, Woodham

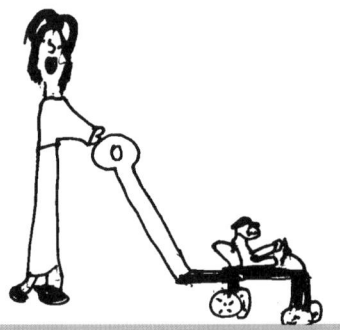

pushchairs: all-terrain

Pegasus Pushchairs Ltd
Westbridge, Tavistock, Devon. 01462 450432

Practical Pushchairs Ltd
Pump Cottage, Wheathold, Wolverton, Hampshire. 0118 9817372

PW Trading Ltd
PO Box 506, St Albans, Herts. 01727 811 221

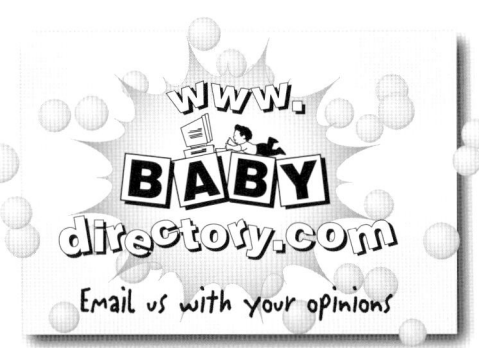

rattles

Plate, Rattle And Bowl
38 Burwood Road, Northampton
01604 406320
www.babies-rattles.co.uk

reflexologists

(see also complementary health)

A gentle treatment that is often used during pregnancy (after 12 weeks) for general relaxation and well being

The British School of Reflexology
01279 429060

British Reflexology Association
01886 821207

Corinne Beveridge
07736 703709

Janet Brophy
01737 351461

TOUCHING LIVES
020 8979 6261
touchinglives@ukgateway.net
See advert on page 53

Camberley
Camberley Natural Therapy Centre
9 Tekels Park
01276 23300
sue@kalicinska.freeserve.co.uk

Dorking
Hilary Lewin
Fairhaven, Radnor Lane, Holmbury, St Mary
01306 730793

Elizabeth Evans
MRSS

Shiatsu practitioner
Reflexologist

Relaxing natural therapies to balance and stimulate the body's own energy flow - beneficial for post and ante-natal care

020 8979 9120

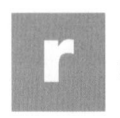

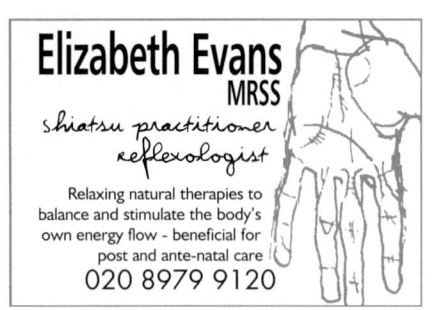

reflexologists (cont.)

Hampton
ELIZABETH EVANS
72 Tangley Park Road. 020 8979 9120
elizabeth.e@tinyworld.co.uk

Isleworth
Sian Smith
54 Thornbury Road. 020 8847 1284

Richmond
Richmond Pharmacy Clinic
82-86 Sheen Road. 020 8940 3930

Twickenham
Linda Arthur
020 8892 2480

Walton-on-Thames
Sally Ann Rees
Lifestyle Natural Health Centre,
4 The Shopping Centre, Hersham Green
01932 254624

Woking
Suzanne Batchelor
11 Highclere Court, Knaphill
01483 486008 / 487198
Batchelor@suzanne999.freeserve.co.uk
www.maternityreflexology.com

registration of births

(see also naming ceremonies)

You have six weeks to decide on "its" name before you must register your baby with your local Registry Office

restaurants: child-friendly

These restaurants usually have high chairs and changing facilities. Some also offer crayons, toys or entertainers at Sunday lunch times. Chains such as Pizza Express and ASK Pizza tend to be child-friendly

Chertsey
The Twynersh House
Thorpe Road. 01932 568231

Esher
Greek Vine
The Green, St Leonards Road, Claygate
01372 465125

The Moore Place
Portsmouth Road. 01372 463532

Godalming
The Manor Inn
Guildford Road. 01483 427134

Guildford
The Worplesdon Place Hotel
Perry Hill, Worplesdon. 01483 232407

Hampton Hill
Joe's Café Bar & Restaurant
99 High Streer. 020 8941 7309

Hounslow
Debenhams Coffee Shop
2nd Floor, Debenhams, Treaty Centre
020 8230 6608

Isleworth
Greedies
South Street. 020 8560 8562

Kew
Browns Restaurant
3-5 Kew Road, Kew Green. 020 8948 4838

Kingston-upon-Thames
TGIF
Bentalls Centre. 020 8547 2900

Wagamamas
16-18 High Street. 020 8546 1117

Redhill
The Mill House
Brighton Road, Salfords. 01737 767277

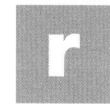

Richmond
Canyon
Riverside. 020 8948 2944

Murano
3 Hill Street. 020 8948 8330

Richmond Harvest
5 The Square. 020 8940 1138
Vegetarian

Teddington
Shambles
83 High Street. 020 8977 9398

Twickenham
Osteria Pulcinella
36 Church Street. 020 8892 5854

O'zon
33 London Road. 020 8891 3611

Woking
The Bridge Barn
Bridge Barn Lane, Horsell. 01483 763642

re-training

Been out of the office for a year or two? Worried that you are hopelessly out of date? Need a refresher course, or just a bit of mental stimulation after all that posseting and nappy talk? Check out Adult Education classes (some offer creches), the Open University, your Local Authority careers advice. Look in local papers, the library, buy a copy of Floodlight (available at newsagents) for all London course listings

riding

Many stables do not recommend riding for under 5s

Chessington
Old Barn Stables
Woodstock Lane South. 020 8398 0822
3yrs+

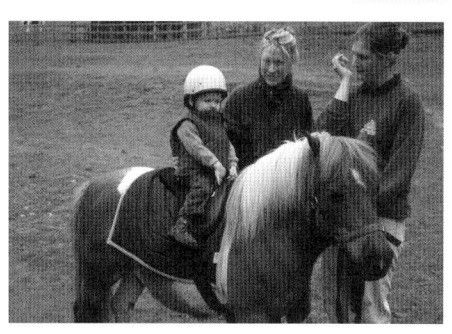

Cobham
Pound Farm Stables
Pound Farm Old Lane. 01932 868652

Kingston-upon-Thames
Kingston Riding Centre
38 Crescent Road. 020 8546 6361

London
Stag Lodge Stables
Robin Hood Gate, Richmond Park
020 8974 6066

Lower Morden
Green Lane Riding Stables
Garth Road. 020 8337 3853

Tadworth
Orchard Cottage Riding Stables
Babylon Lane, Lower Kingswood
01737 241311

Woking
Shey Copse Riding Centre
Maybury. 01483 770022

rocking horses

(see also nursery furniture & decor)

Robert Mullis
01793 813583

safety advice

(see also first aid courses)

Child Accident Prevention Trust (CAPT)
18-20 Farringdon Lane, London, EC1
020 7608 3828

Nannycam
24 Parr Road, London, E6. 020 8471 8616
Hidden camera rental

Safe & Sound
020 8449 8722
info@safe-and-sound.org.uk
www.safe-and-sound.org.uk
Would you or your nanny/au pair know what to do if your child stopped breathing? Ring for first aid courses in your area

school consultants

GABBITAS EDUCATIONAL CONSULTANTS
Carrington House,
126-130 Regent Street, London, W1
020 7734 0161
admin@gabbitas.co.uk
www.gabbitas.com

ISCis London & South-East
Grosvenor Gardens House,
35-37 Grosvenor Gardens, London, SW1
020 7798 1560
southeast@iscis.uk.net
www.iscis.uk.net/southeast

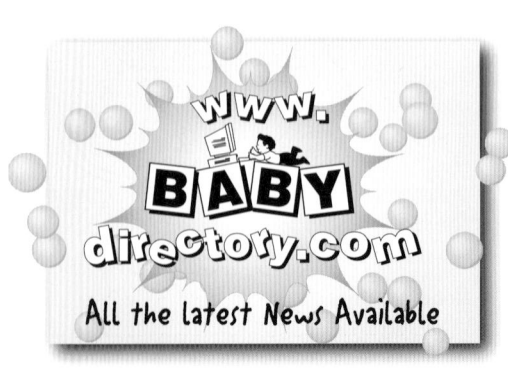

schools: pre-prep

(see also education, nurseries)

For a list of state schools in your area, contact your local council *(see councils)*. ISC or Gabbitas (see above, school consultants) can also supply information on private schools in your area. The following schools have a nursery section

Ashford
St David's Junior School
Church Road. 01784 252494

Ashtead
PARSONS MEAD SCHOOL
Ottways Lane. 01372 276401
www.parsonsmeadsurrey.co.uk
Girls 2½-18yrs

Bagshot
Hall Grove Preparatory School
London Road. 01276 473059
Boys 4-13yrs

Banstead
Greenacre School
Sutton Lane. 01737 352114
Girls 3-18yrs

Priory School
Bolters Lane. 01737 354479
Boys 3-13yrs

Camberley
Clewborough House School
Clewborough Drive. 01276 64799
Co-ed 2-11yrs

Camberley
Hawley Place School
Fernhill Road. 01276 32028
Girls 2-16yrs, boys 2-11yrs

Lyndhurst School
36 The Avenue. 01276 22895
Co-ed 2-12yrs

St Catherine's School
Park Road. 01276 23511
2½-5yrs

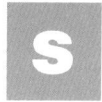

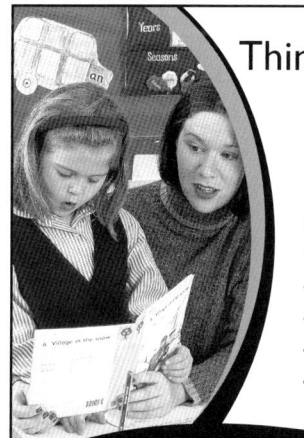

Thinking about independent schools?

Gabbitas offers friendly, independent, expert advice on all stages of your child's education:

- Choosing the right school
- Educational assessment
- Private tutors
- Sixth-form and university education

Call us for a **free** personal selection of independent prep or senior schools suitable for your child

020 7734 0161
www.gabbitas.co.uk

Gabbitas Educational Consultants
126 - 130 Regent Street
London W1B 5EE

Tel: 020 7734 0161
Fax: 020 7437 1764
Email: admin@gabbitas.co.uk

Photograph: The English School, Kuwait

GABBITAS
Educational Consultants

Caterham
Caterham Preparatory School
Harestone Valley Road. 01883 342097
Co-ed 3-11yrs

Oakhyrst Grange School
Stanstead Road. 01883 343344
Boys with some girls 2-12yrs

Chobham
Coworth Park School
Valley End. 01276 855707
Girls with some boys 3-11yrs

Cobham
American Community School
Heywood. 01932 867251
Co-ed 3-18yrs

Feltonfleet School
01932 862264
Co-ed 3-13yrs

Please say you saw the ad in
The Local Baby Directory

'Success Through Excellence'

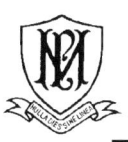

PARSONS MEAD SCHOOL
ASHTEAD

GSA 300 girls aged 2½–18

Enquiries and visits are always welcome

For further details and a prospectus please contact the Admissions Officer:

Telephone:
01372 276401

Fax:
01372 278596

e-mail:
parsonsmead@parsonsmead.co.uk

- Genuine 'added value' through individual attention in small classes
- A caring friendly learning environment
- Excellent results at all levels
- New Learning Support Centre now open
- New Sixth Form Centre opening September
- Flexible Overnight and Day boarding available
- Minibuses now running from Kingston and Surbiton, Ashtead Station and surrounding areas

VISIT OUR WEBSITE AT
www.parsonsmeadsurrey.co.uk
Parsons Mead School, Ottways Lane,
Ashtead, Surrey KT21 2PE

Parsons Mead exists for the furtherance of education Charity no. 312062

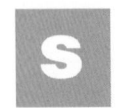

schools: pre-prep (cont.)

Notre Dame Preparatory School
Burwood House. 01932 862152
Girls some boys 3-11yrs

Parkside School
The Manor. 01932 862749
Boys with some girls 2-13yrs

Cranleigh
Duke of Kent School
Ewhurst. 01483 277313
4-13yrs

Croydon
Old Palace School of John Whitgift
Old Palace Road. 020 8688 2027
Girls 4-18yrs

Royal Russell Preparatory School
Coombe Lane. 020 8651 5884
Co-ed 3-11yrs

Dorking
Belmont School
Feldemore. 01306 730852
Co-ed 4-13yrs

Stanway School
Chichester Road. 01306 882151
Girls with some boys 2-11yrs

Englefield Green
Bishopsgate School
01784 432109
Co-ed 2-13yrs

Epsom
Ewell Castle Junior School
Spring Street. 020 8393 3952
Co-ed 3-11yrs

Epsom
Kingswood House School
56 West Hill. 01372 723590
khschool@aol.com
Boys 3-13yrs

St Christopher's
6 Downs Road. 01372 721807
Co-ed 2-7yrs

Esher
Claremont Fan Court School
01372 467841
Co-ed 3-18yrs

Milbourne Lodge Junior School
22 Milbourne Lane. 01372 462781
Boys school with some girls 3-8yrs

Rowan Preparatory School
6 Fitzlan Road. 01372 462627
office@rowan-prep.demon.co.uk
www.rowan-prep.demon.co.uk
Girls 3-11yrs

Farnham
Barfield School
Runfold. 01252 782271
admin@barfieldschool.com
www.barfieldschool.com
Co-ed 3-13yrs

Edgeborough
01252 792495
Co-ed 3-13yrs

Frensham Heights
Rowledge. 01252 792134
Co-ed 3-18yrs

Godalming
Barrow Hills
Witley. 01428 683639
Co-ed 3-13yrs

St Hilary's School
Holloway Hill. 01483 416551
Girls with some boys 2-11yrs

Guildford
Guildford High School for Girls
London Road. 01483 561440
4-18yrs

Visit us at
www.babydirectory.com

Lanesborough School
Maori Road. 01483 880650
Boys 3-13yrs

Longacre School
Shamley Green. 01483 893225
Co-ed 2-11yrs

Rydes Hill Prep.
Rydes Hill House. 01483 563160
Co-ed 3-11yrs

St Catherines's Junior School
01483 894542
Girls 4-11yrs

Tormead School
Cranley Road. 01483 575101
Girls 4-18

Hampton
DENMEAD SCHOOL
41-43 Wensleydale Road. 020 8979 1844
Co-ed 2½-7yrs, boys only 7-13yrs

Twickenham Preparatory School
Beveree. 020 8979 6216
Co-ed 4-13yrs

Haslemere
Haslemere Preparatory School
The Heights. 01428 642350
Boys 4-14yrs

St Ives School
Three Gates Lane. 01428 643734
Girls 3-11yrs

The Royal School
01428 605407
Girls with some boys 2-18yrs

Hindhead
Amesbury
01428 604322
Co-ed 3-13yrs

St Edmund's School
01428 640808
Boys, some girls 2-13yrs

Isleworth
Ashton House School
50-52 Eversley Crescent. 020 8560 3902
Co-ed 3-11yrs

DENMEAD SCHOOL
(Part of the Hampton School Foundation)

41-43 Wensleydale Road
Hampton
Middlesex
TW12 2LP

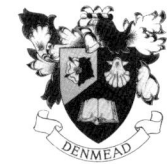

Tel: 020 8979 1844
Fax: 020 8941 8773
Email: denmead@macunlimited.net

Boys 2½ - 13 years   Girls 2½ - 7 years

Common Entrance and Scholarship

- Quality Nursery and Pre-Prep Department
- Wide ranging curriculum within small classes
- Tradition values within a friendly family environment
- Well qualified enthusiastic staff create a caring and industrious environment

Please telephone for a prospectus
I.S.I.S.   Charity No. 312667   I.A.P.S.

Kew
Broomfield House School
10 Broomfield Road. 020 8940 3884
Co-ed 3-11yrs

Kew College
24-26 Cumberland Road. 020 8940 2039
Co-ed 3-11yrs

Unicorn School
238 Kew Road. 020 8948 3926
Co-ed 3-11yrs

Kingston-upon-Thames
Holy Cross Preparatory School
George Road. 020 8942 0729

Park Hill School
8 Queens Road. 020 8546 5496
3-8yrs boys, 3-11yrs girls

Please say you saw the ad in
The Local Baby Directory

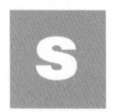

schools: pre-prep (cont.)

Rokeby
George Road. 020 8942 2247
Boys 4-13yrs

Surbiton High School
Surbiton Crescent. 020 8546 5345
Girls with some boys 4-18yrs

Leatherhead
Cranmore School
01483 284137
Boys 3-13yrs

Glennesk School
01483 282329
Co-ed 2-8yrs

St Teresa's Preparatory School
Grove House. 01372 453456
Girls 2-11yrs

Lingfield
Notre Dame School
01342 833176
Co-ed 2-18yrs

Little Bookham
Manor House School
Manor House Lane. 01372 458538
Co-ed 2-16yrs

Long Ditton
Marlborough House Nursery School
Marlborough House. 020 398 6161
0-5yrs

New Malden
Bretby Pre-Prep School
39 Woodlands Avenue. 020 8942 5779

The Study School
57 Thetford Road. 020 8942 0754
Co-ed 3-11yrs

Oxshott
DANES HILL SCHOOL
Leatherhead Road. 01372 842509
www.daneshillschool.co.uk
Co-ed 2½-13yrs

Oxted
Hazelwood School
Wolfs Hill. 01883 712194
Co-ed 3-13yrs

Laverock School
Bluehouse Lane. 01883 714171
Girls 3-11yrs

Purley
Lodge School
Woodcote Road. 020 8660 3179
Girls with some boys 3-18yrs

West Dene School
167 Brighton Road. 020 8660 2404
Co-ed 2-7yrs

Redhill
The Hawthorns
Pendell Court. 01883 743048
office@hawthorns.com
www.hawthorns.com
Co-ed 2-13yrs

Reigate
Dunottar School
High Trees Road. 01737 761945
Girls 3-18yrs

Micklefield School
10-12 Somers Road. 01737 242615
micklefd@globalnet.co.uk
Co-ed 2-11yrs

Reigate St Mary's Preparatory & Choir School
Chart Lane. 01737 244880
www.reigate-stmarys.orh
Co-ed 3-13yrs

Richmond
Kings House
68 Kings Road. 020 8940 7015
Boys 4-13yrs

Visit us at
www.babydirectory.com

INVEST IN EXCELLENCE

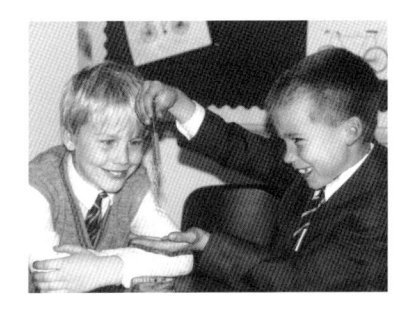

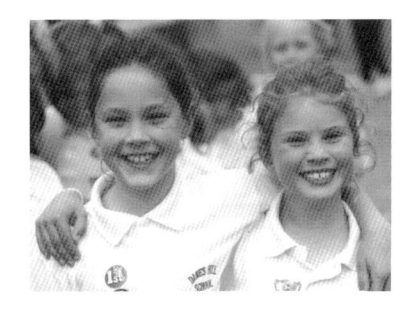

Happy, stimulated girls and boys (aged 2½-13) in a caring and dynamic learning environment.

DANES HILL SCHOOL
Leatherhead Road, Oxshott, Surrey KT22 0JG
(Registrar: 01372 842509)

The Old Vicarage School
48 Richmond Hill. 020 8940 0922
Girls 4-11yrs

South Croydon
Croham Hurst School
79 Croham Road. 020 8680 3064
Girls 3-18yrs, nursery unit

Croydon High School
Old Farleigh Road. 020 8651 5020
Girls 4-18yrs

Cunmore House School
168 Pampisford Road. 020 8660 3445
Co-ed 2-13yrs

Elmhurst School
44-48 South Park Hill Road. 020 8668 0661
Boys 4-11yrs

Sanderstead Junior School
29 Purley Oaks Road. 020 8660 0801
Co-ed 3-11yrs

Staines
Staines Preparatory School
3 Gresham Road. 01784 452916

Sutton
Glaisdale School
14 Arundel Road. 020 8288 1489
Co-ed 3-11yrs

Homefield Preparatory School
Western Road. 020 8642 0965

Seaton House School
67 Banstead Road South. 020 8642 2332

Sutton High School
55 Cheam Road. 020 8642 0594
Girls 4-18yrs

Please say you saw the ad in
The Local Baby Directory

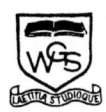

WESTON GREEN SCHOOL

Nursery and Preparatory
020 8398 2778
(Classes from 2 ½ - 8+)

A first class Co-ed Independent School with a fully resourced and active Pre-School

preparing your child to fit into school life by laying solid foundations in the early years.

1. Quality education assured
2. Caring and safe environment
3. Small classes
4. Reasonable fee structure
5. Excellent opportunities for self advancement

Weston Green School
Weston Green Road, Thames Ditton KT7 0JN

---

schools: pre-prep (cOnt.)

Tadworth
Aberdour School
Brighton Road. 01737 354119
Co-ed 3-13yrs

Bramley School
Chequers Lane. 01737 81004
Girls 3-11yrs

Chinthurst School
01737 812011
Boys 3-13yrs

Thames Ditton
WESTON GREEN SCHOOL
Weston Green Road. 020 8398 2778
2½-8yrs. Laying solid foundations in the early years at school

Twickenham
Mall School
185 Hampton Road. 020 8977 2523
Boys 4-13yrs

Newland House School
Waldegrave Park. 020 8892 7479
Boys 4-13yrs

St. Catherine's School
Cross Deep. 020 8891 2898
Girls 3-16yrs

Walton-on-Thames
Danesfield Manor School
Rydens Avenue. 01932 2209300
1-11yrs

WESTWARD SCHOOL
47 Hersham Road. 01932 220911
4-11yrs. Traditional teaching offered by dedicated staff in friendly family school

Weybridge
St George's College Junior School
Weybridge Road. 01932 839300
Co-ed 2-11yrs

Woking
Cable House School
Horsell Rise. 01483 760759

Coworth Park School
Valley End. 01276 855707
Girls with some boys 3-11yrs

Flexlands School
Station Road. 01276 858841
Girls 3-11yrs

Greenfield
Brooklyn Road. 01483 7726525
www.greenfield.surrey.sch.uk

Halstead Preparatory School for Girls
Woodham Rise. 01483 772682
Girls 3-11yrs

Hoe Bridge School
Hoe Place. 01483 760065
Co-ed 2-14yrs

Ripley Court School
Rose Lane. 01483 225217
Co-ed 3-14yrs

St Andrew's School
01483 760943
Co-ed 3-13yrs

Johnsons Shoes

Footwear Specialists

Stockists of:

start-rite — exclusively designed for children

elefanten

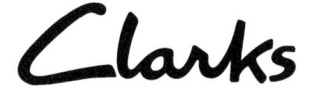

Clarks

·BuCKLe·My·Shoe·

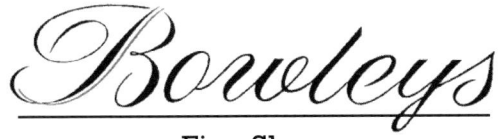

Bowleys

Fine Shoes

sex choice

Materna S.A.
PO Box 21947, London SW3 2ZU
020 7225 3234

shoes

(see also mail order)

BOBUX
07002 466466
www.goo-goo.com
direct@goo-goo.com
Original soft leather shoes for under twos with stayonability!

SHOO SHOOS
Hippychick Ltd, Barford Gables,
Spaxton, Somerset. 01278 671461
sales@hippychickltd.co.uk
www.hippychickltd.co.uk
Imaginative and refreshingly different, soft leather baby shoes (0-24 months)

shoe shops

Ashford
JOHNSONS SHOES
1-2 New Parade. 01784 253137

Bookham
Petits Pieds
7 Grove Corner, Lower Shott. 01372 458585

Carshalton
The Start Rite Shop
60 High Street

Cobham
Shortlands Shoes
21 High Street

Epsom
Best Feet First
9 Spread Eagle Walk. 01372 745353

Please say you saw the ad in
The Local Baby Directory

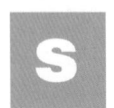

shoe shops (cont.)

Kew
The Shoe Station
3 Station Approach. 020 8940 9905

New Malden
JOHNSONS SHOES
125-129 High Street. 020 8942 3255

Richmond
BOWLEYS
72-73 George Street. 020 8940 1564

PICCOLO BELLA
6 Eton Street. 020 8948 8601
thetoy-station.com
Children's wear 0-6yrs. Dressing up clothes and accessories. Toys and books

Teddington
JOHNSONS SHOES
60-62 Broad Street. 020 8977 4447

Twickenham
JOHNSONS SHOES
37-39 King Street Parade. 020 8892 9012

Walton-on-Thames
JOHNSONS SHOES
28 High Street. 01932 224626

shopping crèches

Kingston-upon-Thames
World Of Children Playcare Centre
Bentalls Centre. 020 8974 8502
1-8yrs

Woking
Stay "N" Play
within Sainsbury's Superstore. 01483 474750
Max. stay 3 hours

single parents

(see also helplines)

Gingerbread
020 7488 9300

Kids No Object
Lymington, Farwell Avenue, Eastergate, Chichester, West Sussex. 01243 543685

Single Parent Travel Club
0870 241 6210

ski companies specialising in children

Chilly Powder
020 7289 6958

Mark Warner
08708 480 482

Meriski
01451 843100

Simply Ski
020 8541 2207

Ski Beat
01243 780405

Ski Company
01451 843123

Ski Famille
01223 363777

Ski Olympic
01709 579999

Ski Scott Dunn
020 8767 0202

Ski Solutions
020 7471 7733

Snowbizz Vacances
01778 341455

ski wear

Discount Kids Ski Gear
01985 850747

Ski Market
020 8741 7037
Second hand and new, 2 yrs+

Ski Occasions
020 8368 1212

Ski Togs
020 8993 9883

Ski Wear Service
020 7435 0124
Buy or sell

skincare

(see also baby toiletries)

E45 JUNIOR
Available from all leading supermarkets and pharmacies
www.e45.com
Dermatologist and paediatrician approved. Developed for children with dry, sensitive skin or eczema

---

Does your child have a sleep problem?

Do you need a good night's sleep?

Children's Sleep Clinic

For professional, tailor-made advice and solutions that work, contact Millpond - specialists, experienced in children's sleep problems.

MILLPOND
bringing harmony

Tel: 020 8941 6370
E-mail: forinfo@mill-pond.co.uk

sleep

Good Sleep Guide for You and Your Baby
PO Box 5868, Forres, IV36 1WH
07020 922750

MILLPOND
020 8941 6370
www.mill-pond.co.uk
forinfo@mill-pond.co.uk
Specialists in children's sleep problems

NIGHT NANNIES
Seven Acres, Church Hill,
Binfield, Berks
01344 862973
iona@night-nannies.com
See advert under nanny agency

Please say you saw the ad in
The Local Baby Directory

sleeping bags

BONNE NUIT
020 8871 1472
sales@bonne-nuit.co.uk
www.bonne-nuit.co.uk
Beautiful French baby sleeping bags available in 3 sizes (0-4 years). Winter & summer collection. Call for brochure or stockist, or order online

Clair de Lune
Shentonfield Road, Wythenshawe, Manchester
0161 491 9800

slimming

Numbers are central information lines. Call for details of your local class

Rosemary Conley Diet and Fitness Clubs
01509 620222

Lighten Up
020 8241 2323

Slimming World
01773 521111

Weight Watchers
08457 123000

spanish

El Club Espanol
020 977 8967

French & Spanish A La Carte
020 8946 4777

speech therapists

Bookham
Say & Play Pre School Groups
Edenside Clinic, 33 Edenside Road
01372 450472

Leatherhead
Speech & Language Therapy Services
Orchard End. 01483 282130

London
Speech, Language and Hearing Centre
1-5 Christopher Place, Chalton Street, NW11
020 7383 3834
www.speech-lang.org.uk
Specialist centre for babies/toddlers with hearing or speech impairment

New Malden
Malden Speech & Language Clinic
17 Selwyn Road. 020 8942 1742

sun protection

SPOSH
07002 466 466
direct@goo-goo.com
www.goo-goo.com
Original UPF50+ swimwear to beat the sun but still have fun!

swimming classes

(see also swimming pools)

Local swimming pools often run classes for aqua-natal, babies and young children

AQUA TOTS BABY SWIMMING
020 8688 6488
evy@aquatots.com
www.aquatots.com
Swimming the natural way, without bouyancy aids. 0-4yrs

Visit us at
www.babydirectory.com

www.babydirectory.com   The Local Baby Directory - *Surrey & S. Middlesex* **Page 113**

Please say you saw the ad in
The Local Baby Directory

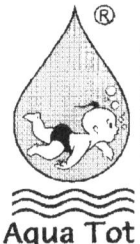

little dippers
infant water safety training

As seen on BBC1's *"Human Body"* series, Channel 4's *"Baby it's you"* and ITV's *"How do they do that"*

It's great fun and could one day save your child's life

For info on local classes call
0870 758 0302

BABY SWIMMING
Swimming the natural way, without the use of bouyancy aids, for 0 - 4 years old. Surrey, Kent & London. Warm pools, small classes, in-pool instructor. Term start in Jan, April, July & Sept.

020 8688 6488
www.aquatots.com

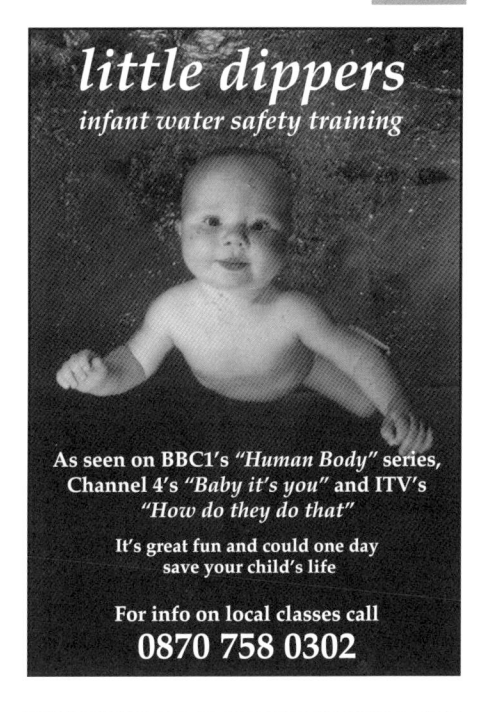

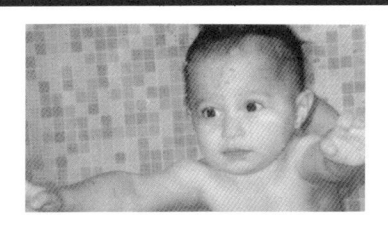

Aqua Tot
~naturally~

BABY
SWIMMING
UNDERWATER SWIMMING
BABIES & TODDLERS
WARM PRIVATE POOLS
SMALL CLASSES/CALL
01865771397

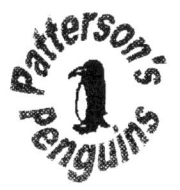

Patterson's penguins
SWIMMING SCHOOL

Fully qualified, experienced teachers - small groups,
Non-swimmers groups (Max 4),
from 6 months to adults.

Holiday 5 day crash courses available.
All abilities from beginners to club level,
Stroke Technique/Diving/
Rookie Lifesaving/Snorkelling.

At private pools in Leatherhead & Twickenham
For further information/Bookings
Phone Guy or Ruth

01372 210999 / 07801 482767

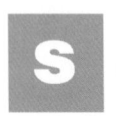

swimming classes (cont.)

BABY SWIMMING
01865 771397/07989 642465
Walton-on-Thames, Guildford & Godalming
See advert on page 113

DOLPHIN SWIM SCHOOLS
020 8640 4488
Own pool with baby classes from 10 wks

LITTLE DIPPERS
0870 7580302
info@littledippers.co.uk
See advert on page 113

PATTERSON'S PENGUINS SWIMMING LESSONS
01372 210999
See advert on page 113

Atlantis Swim School
020 8296 8422
18mths+

Charlotte's Swimming School
01932 788506

Little Dolphins
020 8640 7232

Penguin Swim School
020 8395 7814
Sutton, Kingston, Surbiton, Epsom & Ham

Swim Schools
020 8241 7010/0771 8756030

Swimwise
01372 815905

Water Nippers
01825 767176

Waterbabies
020 8874 6013
Morden & Mitcham

Wilson's School
01737 350503
Ashtead, Epsom & Wallington

swimming pools

(see also health clubs with crèches, leisure centres)

Brentford
BRENTFORD FOUNTAIN
658 Chiswick High Road. 020 8994 9596

Chiswick
NEW CHISWICK POOL
020 8747 8811

Croydon
New Addington Swimming Pool
Central Parade. 01689 842553

Royal Russel Swimming Pool
Coombe Lane. 020 8657 0150
Memebership scheme

East Molesey
Hurst Pool
off Hurst Road. 020 8941 6544

Feltham
FELTHAM AIRPARCS LEISURE CENTRE
020 8894 9156

Haslemere
Herons Swimming & Fitness Centre
Kings Road. 01428 658484

Heston
HESTON POOL
020 8570 4396

Isleworth
ISLEWORTH RECREATION CENTRE
Twickenham Road. 020 8560 6855

Morden
Morden Park Pool
London Road. 020 8640 6727

Richmond
Pools on the Park
Old Deer Park, Twickenham Road, Richmond
020 8940 0561

Teddington
Teddington Pool
Vicarage Road. 020 8977 9911

Walton-On-Thames
Walton Swimming Pool
Kings Close. 01932 222984

Let Hounslow teach you to Swim

Our Swim Development Scheme has been carefully & professionally designed to provide a full range of classes to suit all abilities and ages from beginners through to advanced swimmers.

**Courses start in January, April and September
Call now for more details**

Brentford Fountain Leisure Centre ... Tel: 020 8994 - 9596
Feltham Airparcs Leisure Centre ... Tel: 020 8894 - 9156
Isleworth Recreation Centre ... Tel: 020 8560 - 6755
Heston Pool ... Tel: 020 8570 - 4396
New Chiswick Pool ... Tel: 020 8747 - 8811

WORKING IN PARTNERSHIP WITH HOUNSLOW

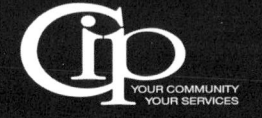

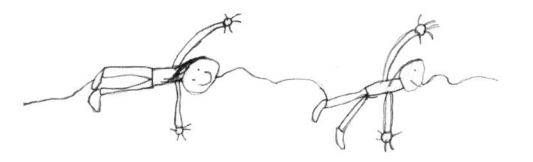

Further away, but worth the trip:

Coral Reef
Nine Mile Ride, Bracknell, Berks. 01344 862525

Aquasplash
Leisure World, Jarman Park, Hemel Hempstead, Herts. 01442 292203
"This swimming pool is great for people who like getting their face wet unlike my mum. There are six slides. I give this pool 10/10." Hannah Levy

swimming pools: outdoor

Usually only open during the summer months

Addlestone
Abbeylands Sports Centre
School Lane. 01932 858966

Guildford
Guildford Lido
Stoke Road. 01483 444888

Hampton
Hampton Open Air Pool
High Street. 020 8255 1116

Richmond
Pools on the Park
Old Deer Park. 020 8940 0561

Please say you saw the ad in
The Local Baby Directory

tennis

Also check out your local leisure centre

Will to Win Tennis Centre
020 8994 1466
www.tennis-uk.com
Chiswick House grounds. Also Holland Park and Ealing. Coaching and play from 3-10yrs. Women's drop-in tennis mornings

TENS machines

Pain relief without drugs. Also available through the NCT

Concept Group
020 8941 6652

Trust Tens
020 9546 1616

theatres

(see also arts centres, drama)

Many theatres stage shows for children, especially around Christmas

Artsline
London's information and advice service for disabled people on arts & entertainment.
020 7388 2227
Also produce a booklet caled 'Play' on activities for disabled children (£2)

Puppet Theatre Barge
020 7249 6876
Varying locations throughout the year

Brentford
Watermans Art Centre
40 High Street. 020 8232 1010
Pantomimes and regular childrens shows

Croydon
Warehouse Theatre
Dingwall Road. 020 8681 1257

Hounslow
Paul Robeson Theatre
Treaty Centre, High Street. 020 8577 6969

Redhill
Harlequin Theatre
Warwick Quadrant. 01737 765547

Richmond
Richmond Theatre
The Green. 020 8940 0088
Pantomines

Walton-on-Thames
Riverhouse Barn
Manor Road. 01932 253354

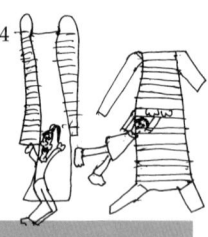

theme parks

Alton Towers
Staffordshire. 0870 520 4060

Chessington World of Adventure
Surrey. 01372 727227

Disneyland
Marne-la-Vallee Cedex 4, France
0870 50 30 303

Efteling
Europalaan 1, Kaasheuvel, Netherlands
00-31-41 62288 111
Dutch theme park

Legoland
Berkshire. 01753 626100

Thorpe Park
Surrey. 0932 562633

toy libraries

Early Learning Centres have Tuesday morning 'open days' - play time and activities (check with individual branches for times)

National Association of Toy and Leisure Libraries
68 Churchway, NW1. 020 7387 9592
SAE for list of closest toy library

toy shops

(see also mail order: toys)

Early Learning Centre and Mothercare have branches on many high streets, along with Toys 'R' Us

Bagshot
Jack-In-The-Box
49 High Street. 01276 473805

Carshalton
JH Lorimer
77 Banstead Road. 020 8642 1099

Cobham
Funtasia
Oakdene Parade. 01932 867374

Coulsdon
JH Lorimer
140 Brighton Road. 020 8668 9186

Croydon
Gordon's Toys & Stationary
255a Lower Addiscombe Road. 020 8654 5015

Ewell Village
Mobo's Toy Box
73 High Street. 020 8873 7210

Guildford
The Bear Garden & Dolls Attic
10 Jeffries Passage. 01483 302581

Enchanted Wood
3-5 Kings Road, Shalford. 01483 570088

LITTLE WONDERS
12 Angel Gate. 01483 577648
www.littlewonders.co.uk
See advert on page 118

Hampton Court
Zebedees
8 Bridge Road. 020 8979 2979

Lingfield
Lingfield Rocking Horses
High Street. 01342 836684
Wooden toys

Morden
TST Outdoor Toys
47 St Helier Avenue. 020 8640 1195

Oxted
JH Lorimer
86-88 Station Road East. 01883 715305

Purley
JH Lorimer
934 Brighton Road. 020 8660 9716

Redhill
Gamleys
38 The Belfrey Centre, Station Road
01737 773941

Reigate
Reigate Toys & Models
7 Western Parade. 01737 245313

Richmond
The Farmyard
54 Friars Stile Road. 020 8332 0038

PICCOLO BELLA
6 Eton Street. 020 8948 8601
www.thetoy-station.com
Children's wear 0-6yrs. Dressing up clothes and accessories. Toys and books

Toy Station
10 Eton Street. 020 8940 4896

Tridias
Litchfield Terrace, Sheen Road. 020 8948 3459

Stanwell
Toys Plus
59 Clare Road. 01784 257249

toy shops (cont.)

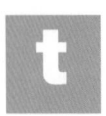

Surbiton
CHILDHOOD DISCOVERIES
23 Victoria Road. 020 8390 2168
www.educational-toys.co.uk

Sutton
Gamleys
St Nicholas Centre, St Nicholas Way
020 8770 3532

Jigsaw Gallery
Unit 23, Level One Stt Nicholas Centre,
St Nicholas Way. 020 8661 7597

Teddington
Pinocchio Gifts
79 High Street. 020 8977 8995
www.pinocchio-bearstore.com

PLAY INSIDE OUT
42 Broad Street. 020 8614 5628
info@playinsideout.com

Twickenham
LITTLE WONDERS
3 York Street. 020 8255 6114
www.littlewonders.co.uk

Papillon Toy Shop
37 Church Street. 020 8892 5637

Walton-on-Thames
Hankards
103 New Zealand Avenue. 01932 227017

Whitton
Papillon Toy Shop
87 High Street. 020 8755 1870

Worcester Park
Household & Toy Warehouse
103 Central Road. 020 8337 0727

Windlesham
Rainbow Play Systems
Hillier Garden Centres, London Road
01344 874662
Climbing frames

Little Wonders

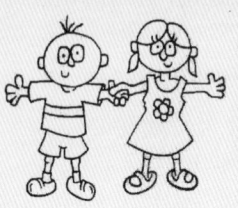

Sevi, Plan Toys, Lucy Locket, Ty, Jellycat, Bobux, Le Toy Van, Manhattan Toys, Siku, Galt
And many many more.

The Best in Quality Toys & Gifts.

Come and see our Fantastic range of Fun Games, Dolls Houses, Baby Toys, Madeline, Bead Frames, Educational Games and Gifts with a Difference.

3 York Street, Twickenham
12 Angel Gate Guildford or
Visit our Web Site: www.littlewonders.co.uk
For secure on line shopping

Childhood Discoveries

"Where all the best toys are hiding"

Wooden Toys ~ Castles, Dolls' Houses, Thomas Railway, Garages, Farms and Ride-on toys.

Other areas include ~
Art & Craft, Puppets & Theatre, Puzzles, Games, Science & Nature, Outdoor Play Equipment, Books, Tapes and much, much more.

Visit us at
www.educational-toys.co.uk
23 Victoria Road, Surbiton, Surrey, KT6 4JZ
020-8390-2168

PLAY INSIDE OUT
LEARNING THROUGH PLAY
Educational Play Specialists
0-11 years+

offering individual advice on:
Toys, Play Equipment, Games, CD Roms, Puzzles, Books

an outdoor range including:
Swings, Slides, Sandboxes, Trampolines, Wooden Playhouses and Treehouses

and

An Outdoor Play Area Advice/Design Service

plus

Support and Learning Materials for School Curriculum Events, Gift Vouchers Available

42 Broad Street, Teddington, TW11 8QY
Tel: 020 8614 5628
Fax: 020 8614 5669
email: info@playinsideout.com

travel with kids

There are Baby Directory guides to great swathes of the UK. See our order form at the beginning of the book, or check out our website at **www.babydirectory.com**
Here are some other publications and websites

Edinburgh for Under Fives

Kids Gids
Guide to Amsterdam

Le Paris des tout-petits
Guide to Paris

www.babygoes2.co
01273 230669

www.travellingwithchildren.co.uk
01684 594831

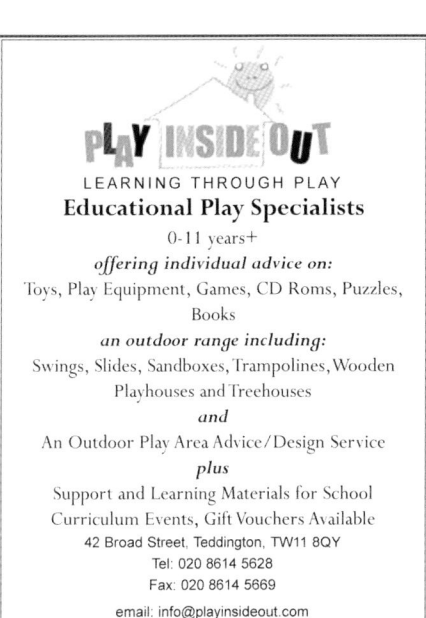

travel companies specialising in children

(see also ski companies, travel with kids)

The Bosman Safari Company
07880 732115

Club Med
106 Brompton Road, London, SW3
020 7581 1161
Brochures: 01455 852 202

Eurocamp
0870 9019 451

EuroVillages
01606 787776

Mark Warner
0870 848 0482

tuition

Fleet Tutors
24 Northfield Road, Church Cookham
01252 812262
support@fleet-tutors.co.uk
www.fleet-tutors.co.uk

twins

(see also helplines: multiple births)

Twins and Multiple Births Association (TAMBA)
0151 3480 020
Contact for help, support and details of your local group organiser

Croydon & District Twins Club
020 8645 9470

Please say you saw the ad in
The Local Baby Directory

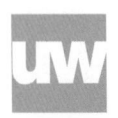

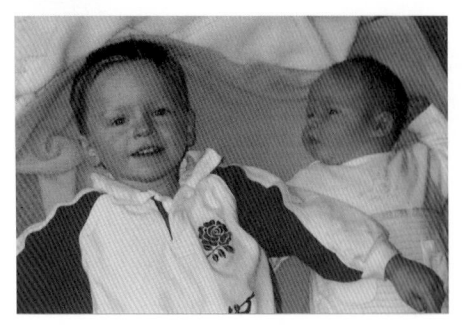

under 5's centres

Also known as one o'clock clubs. A wonderful invention! Open usually Monday-Friday, 1-4pm, maybe longer on holidays, one o'clock clubs provide painting equipment, trikes, water play, balls, etc in addition to basic playground equipment. There is usually an indoor and an outdoor section.

Kingston-upon-Thames
Toddlers Fun Time
The Hawker Centre, Lower Ham Road
020 8296 9747
1-5yrs
Wed, 10-12pm, 12.30-2.30pm. Fri 10-2pm

Twickenham
Marble Hill Park
Marble Hill Park, Richmond Road, Twickenham. 020 8891 0641
Small charge

The UK's longest established Birthing Tub Hire Company - attractive tubs with heater units and water maintenance kits to keep the water warm, clean & clear and ready to use at a moment's notice, giving a natural pain relief.

Phone: 020 8568 4913
www.birthworks.co.uk

---

vaccinations

Try talking to your health visitor, G.P., homeopath or contacting the following organisations

Direct Health 2000
6-7 Grove Market Place, Court Yard, London
0870 443 7070

Informed Parent
020 8861 1022
Information

JABS
01942 713565

NHS Direct
0845 4647

Westminster & Pimlico Medical Centre
15 Denbigh Street, London. 020 7834 6969

www.immunisation.org.uk
020 7972 3807

water births

If planning a hospital delivery, check with your local hospital for their facilities and policies on water birth (see hospitals: NHS, hospitals, private)

BIRTHWORKS
020 8568 4913

Splashdown
0870 44 44 403

water exercise in pregnancy

Many local swimming pools run aqua-natal courses (see swimming pools)

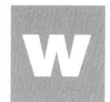

web sites

www.babydirectory.com

Directory, bookshop, encyclopaedia, nanny agency, links to thousands of other baby/child related companies…

working opportunities

KATE WOOD, COMPLEMENTARY HEALTH PRODUCTS
020 8608 1857
kateandchris@blueyonder.co.uk
Seeking enthusiastic, motivated individuals for genuinely exciting opportunity. Part-time cash or full-time career!

Brainworks Direct
020 8891 2588
Educational software sales

Interactive Kids
020 8891 1644
alayne@interactive-kids.co.uk

jo jingles
01494 676575
Music groups for pre schoolers

SING AND SIGN
01273 550587
www.singandsign.com
Run your own music groups teaching established baby signing programme

Usborne Books at Home
5 Swift Close, Uckfield. 01825 769515

Working Options
14-16 Hamilton Road, W5. 020 8932 1462
www.working-options.co.uk
Part time professional recruitment

Please say you saw the ad in **The Local Baby Directory**

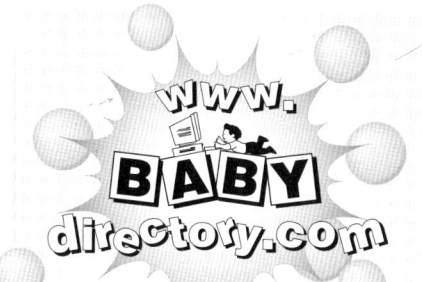

---

www.babydirectory.com

Come and visit us

- Over 40,00 local listings
- Encyclopaedia of Pregnancy & Birth
- Medical Advice ■ Breastfeeding
- Educational Advice
- Nanny Agency
- Book Shop ■ Prizes ■ Updates

Make your life easier

Sing and Sign

An exciting new concept!

Teach baby signing the fun way
Baby music groups with a difference!

With action-songs and nursery rhymes, Sing and Sign teaches simple signing for hearing babies, enabling communication before speech

If you can sing in tune and have a lively personality you could
Run your own Sing and Sign classes

Flexible hours
Comprehensive training
Ongoing support
Lesson plans
Own area
Low start-up cost/high returns

Learn more about us
visit www.singandsign.com
Call for an information pack **01273-550587**

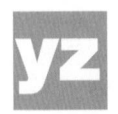

yoga in pregnancy or for children

(see also antenatal teachers)

British Wheel of Yoga
01529 306851
Contact for list of teachers

Garry Freer
020 8408 4121
garryfreer@blueyonder.co.uk

Yoga in Pregnancy
020 8892 3439

New Malden
Ruth Armes
020 8395 9435

Sunbury
Pia Harris
01784 254508

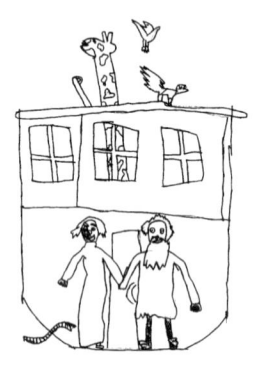

zoos

(see also farms, outings, parks & playgrounds)

Bedfordshire
Whipsnade Wild Animal Park
Whipsnade, nr Dunstable. 01582 872171

Woburn Safari Park
Woburn. 01525 290407
Drive-through wildlife park. M1 Jct 12 or 13

East Sussex
Drusilla's Park
Alfriston. 01323 874100
One mile N of Alfriston, on A27 between Eastbourne & Brighton

Hampshire
Marwell Zoological Park
Colden Common, Winchester. 01962 777407
B2177, 6 miles sough of Winchester from Jct 11, M3

Hertfordshire
Paradise Wildlife Park
White Stubbs Lane, Broxbourne. 01992 470490

London
Battersea Park Zoo
North Carriage Drive
Monkeys, cow, smaller mammals, kangaroos. Poor café

London Zoo
Regents Park. 020 7722 3333
The works

Oxfordshire
Cotswold Wildlife Park
Burford. 01993 823006
On A361. 120 acres, rhinos, etc

Surrey
Birdworld and Underwater World
Holt Pound, Farnham. 01420 22140
Spring/summer opening

British Wildlife Centre
Gate House Farm, Newchapel. 01342 834658
Host children's birthday parties

Gatwick Zoo
Russ Hill. 01293 8623120

Visit us at
www.babydirectory.com

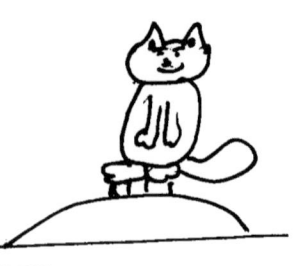

index

Italic categories cross-refer to additional entries; roman type refers readers to the main entries elsewhere

a pages 1-5

accessories see clothing shops, linens, mail order, nearly new, shoe shops
acupuncture
 see also complementary health
ADD see helplines - hyperactivity
adventure playgrounds
 see also indoor adventure playcentres, parks & playgrounds
advice see helplines, nursery advisory services
after school clubs
AIDS see helplines
alexander technique
 see also exercise classes personal trainers
allergies see helplines
all-terrain buggies see pushchairs
alternative health see complementary health,
 see also acupuncture, homoeopathy, massage, osteopaths
amsterdam see travel with kids
anaphylaxis see helplines
antenatal support & information
 see also helplines, hospitals, midwives
antenatal teachers
 see also antenatal support & information
antenatal testing
aquanatal see swimming classes, swimming pools
aquaria see outings
arabic
aromatherapy:
 see also baby toiletries, complementary health, massage
 mail order
 aromatherapists
art
 see also ceramics, dance, drama, music
arts centres see theatres
asthma see helplines
astrological charts

au pair agencies
 see also babysitters, childminders, nanny agencies
autism see helplines

b pages 6-10

baby equipment see nursery goods
baby research
baby toiletries
baby sleeping bags see linens
babysitters
 see also childminders, nanny agencies
back carriers see carriers
back problems see osteopaths, physiotherapists
ballet see dance
balloons see party equipment
beauty treatments see baby toiletries, complementary health
bedwetting see helplines
benefits
bereavement see helplines
bicycles see cycling
birth see antenatal support, antenatal teachers, helplines, hospitals, midwives,
birth announcements
 see also cards
birthday cakes see cakes
birthing pools see water births
birth support
 see antenatal support & information, doulas, hospitals, midwives, TENS, waterbirth
blindness see helplines
body painter
book clubs for children
book shops for children
bouncy castles see indoor adventure playcentres; for rental see party equipment
brain injury see helplines
bras see maternity wear
breastfeeding
 accessories
 advice
 see also maternity wear
buggies, all-terrain see pushchairs
buggy repair see pram & buggy repair
bullying see helplines

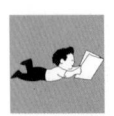

INDEX The Local Baby Directory - Surrey & S. Middlesex www.babydirectory.com

c — pages 11-18

caesarians see helplines
cakes
  see also party catering
car seats & accessories
  see also nursery goods
cards
  see also birth announcements
carriers
cassettes & CDs
castings
CDs see cassettes & CDs
cerebral palsy
  see also helplines
ceramics
chemists: late opening
chess
childcare listings magazine
children's savings see financial advice
childminders
  see also au pair agencies, babysitters, nanny agencies
chiropractic
christening gowns
cinemas
cleaners
cleft lip see helplines
climbing frames see toys
clinics
clothing shops
  see also mail order, maternity wear, nearly new shops, nursery goods, shoe shops
clubs
  see also after school clubs
coeliac disease see helplines
complementary health:
  see also acupuncture, aromatherapy, homeopathy, massage, osteopathy, reflexology, yoga
computers for children
concerts
contraception see family planning
cookery
cot death see helplines
cots see cradles, nursery furniture & decor
councils
cradles
  see also nursery furniture & decor
craniosacral therapy

crèches see nurseries
crèches, for shopping see shopping crèches
crèches: mobile
cruelty see helplines
crying see helplines
cycling & cycling attachments
cystic fibrosis see helplines

d — pages 19-21

dance
  see also art, drama, gym, music
deafness see helplines
death see helplines
dentists
designers
designer outlets
diabetes see helplines
diet see slimming
disability see helplines
divorce see helplines
dolls' hospitals see hospitals
dolls' houses
  see also toy shops
doulas
down's syndrome see helplines
drama
  see also art, dance, gym, music, theatres
dressing up see fancy dress
drop-in see clinics, under 5's centres parent & toddler groups
dyslexia see helplines, learning difficulties
dyspraxia see helplines

e — page 22

eczema see helplines
education see educational consultants, helplines, nurseries, schools, tuition
educational consultants
  see also helplines: education, schools, tuition
educational organisations see helplines: education, schools, tuition
entertainers see party entertainers
enuresis see bedwetting
epilepsy see helplines

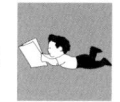

www.babydirectory.com   The Local Baby Directory - *Surrey & S. Middlesex*   **INDEX**

equipment see hiring, nearly new, nursery goods, pushchairs
equipment hire see hiring, party equipment
exercise classes for ante- & post-natal
see also antenatal support, gym, health clubs, leisure centres, personal trainers, physiotherapists, swimming pools, yoga
ex-pat advice
eyes

f   pages 23-26

face painting see party entertainers
family planning
fancy dress:
   mail order
   retail
farms
see also parks & playgrounds, outings, zoos
fatherhood
see also helplines
feeding bras see breastfeeding accessories
fertility see infertility
feng shui
financial advice
first aid courses
fitness see exercise, health clubs, leisure centres, swimming pools
flower remedies
folic acid see nutrition
food:
see also organic, pubs, restaurants
football
see also leisure centres
footprints
see also ceramics
formula milk see helplines
fragile X see helplines
french classes & clubs:
   language aids

g   pages 27-29

german classes & clubs
gifted children
see also helplines
gifts
see also mail order
godchildren see gifts

GP see helplines, health
growth see helplines
gym
see also indoor adventure playcentres, leisure centres

h   pages 30-42

hairdressers
health see helplines
health clubs with crèches
see also exercise, leisure centres, personal trainers, swimming pools
healthfood shops
see also organic
helplines
herpes see helplines
high chairs see nursery furniture, nursery goods
hiring equipment
see also nearly new shops, party equipment
HIV see helplines: aids
holiday play schemes
holidays see hotels and holidays, ski travel, travel companies
home birth
see also antenatal support& information, midwives
home delivery services
   babies see midwives
   nappies see nappy delivery, nappy laundry
home education see helplines, tuition
homeopathy
see also complementary health
hospitals
   dolls & teddies
   NHS
   private maternity
hotels & holidays
hyperactivity see helplines
hypnosis see hypnotherapy
hypnotherapy

i   page 43-44

ice rinks
indoor adventure playcentres
infertility
internet
see also websites

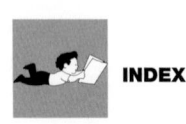

INDEX The Local Baby Directory - *Surrey & S. Middlesex* — www.babydirectory.com

l   pages 44-48

learning difficulties
  see also helplines
left-handedness
legal advice
leisure centres
  see also health clubs with crèches, swimming pools
libraries
  see also toy libraries
lice
linens
  see also sleeping bags

m   pages 49-59

magazines
mail order:
  see also aromatherapy, fancy dress, gifts, home delivery, linens, maternity wear, organic, sleeping bags
  accessories
  baby goods
  clothing
  gifts
  nursery goods
  shoes
  toys
manufacturers & suppliers
marriage *see helplines*
martial arts
massage for baby & mother
maternity benefits *see benefits*
maternity bras *see breastfeeding accessories, maternity wear*
maternity nannies
  see also midwives, nanny agencies
maternity services *see helplines, hospitals*
maternity wear:
  mail order
  retail
mathematics
ME *see helplines*
meditation
meningitis *see helplines*
mental stimulation *see re-training*
midwives: independent
  see also antenatal support & information, maternity nannies
miscarriage *see helplines*
montessori *see nurseries*
motherhood *see helplines*
mother's helps *see au pair agencies, babysitters, cleaners, childminders, nanny agencies*
multiple births *see helplines: twins*
murals & painted nursery furniture
  see also nursery furniture & decor, nursery goods
museums
  see also outings
music
  see also art, dance, drama

n   pages 60-86

name tapes
naming ceremonies
  see also registration of births
nanny agencies
  see also au pair agencies, babysitters, childminders, maternity nannies & nurses
nanny payroll services
  see also financial advice
nanny tax advice *see nanny payroll services*
nappies, cloth & other
nappy information
nappy delivery, hire & laundry
natural products
  see also complementary health, organics
nature reserves
  see also farms, parks & playgrounds
naturopaths
  see complementary health, osteopaths
nearly new equipment, toy & clothing shops
nits *see lice*
nurses *see maternity nannies, medical advice, midwives*
nurseries: private & nursery schools
  see also education, schools, tuition
nursery furniture & decor
  see also murals, nursery goods
nursery goods
  see also clothing shops, mail order, murals & painted furniture, nearly new, nursery furniture & decor
nursery schools *see nurseries*
nutrition

www.babydirectory.com   The Local Baby Directory - *Surrey & S. Middlesex*   **INDEX**

o   pages 86-89

organic
see also food, health food shops, nappies, cloth & other
osteopaths
see also craniosacral therapy
outdoor play see parks & playgrounds
outings
see also farms, indoor adventure playcentres, museums, parks & playgrounds, theatres, theme parks, zoos

p   pages 90-99

parent & toddler groups
parentcraft classes & advice
paris see travel with kids
parks & playgrounds
see also adventure playgrounds, outings
parenthood see helplines
party entertainers
party equipment:
see also fancy dress, party entertainers
  mail order
  retail
party venues
paternity testing
personal trainers
see also exercise classes, health clubs
photographers
  specialising in babies & children
physiotherapists
play see indoor adventure playcentres, parks & playgrounds
playcentres see indoor adventure playcentres, under 5's centres
playgrounds see adventure playgrounds, parks & playgrounds
playgroups
postnatal depression see helplines
postnatal groups see mother & baby groups
postnatal support & information
see also breastfeeding, helplines: postnatal advice
pram & buggy repairs
prams see pushchairs, nursery goods
pre-eclampsia see helplines

pregnancy testing
private education see nurseries, schools
psychologists & psychotherapists
pubs with gardens or playrooms
puppets see party entertainers
pushchairs:, all-terrain
pyjamas see linens

r   pages 99-101

rainy day activities see indoor adventure playcentres, museums
rattles
recruitment see working opportunities
reflexologists
see also complementary health
registration of births
see also naming ceremonies
reiki see complementary health
rental see hiring, party equipment
repair see hospitals: dolls & teddies, pram & buggy repair
restaurants: child-friendly
retraining
returning to work see helplines: work, re-training, working opportunities
riding
rocking horses
see also nursery furniture & decor

s   pages 102-115

safety advice
school consultants
school fees see financial advice
schools: pre-prep
see also education, nurseries
second hand see nearly new
sex choice
sexual abuse see helplines
shiatsu see massage
shoes
see also mail order
shoe shops
shopping crèches

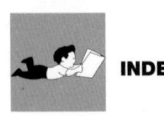

INDEX The Local Baby Directory - *Surrey & S. Middlesex* www.babydirectory.com

sick children see hospitals
single parents
 see also helplines
skating see ice rinks
ski companies specialising in children
ski wear
skincare
 see also baby toiletries
sleep
sleeping bags see linens
slimming
slings see carriers
smoking see helplines
spanish
speech therapists
spina bifida see helplines
sports centres see leisure centres, swimming pools
stammering see helplines
summer camps see holiday playschemes
sun protection
swimming classes
 see also swimming pools
swimming pools:
 see also health clubs, leisure centres
 indoor
 outdoor

t pages 116-119

tennis
TENS machines
termination see helplines
theatres
 see also arts centres, drama
theme parks
toddler groups see mother & baby groups
toiletries see baby toiletries
toy libraries
toy repairs see hospitals: doll & teddies
toy shops
 see also mail order: toys
training see re-training
trains see outings

travel companies specialising in children
 see also ski companies, travel with kids
travel with kids
tuition
twins
 see also helplines: multiple births

u page 120

under 5's centres

v page 120

vaccinations
violence See helplines

w pages 120-121

water births
water exercise in pregnancy
web sites
wills see helplines
work see helplines
working opportunities
widowhood see helplines

y page 122

yoga in pregnancy or for children
 see also antenal teachers

z page 122

zoos
 see also farms, outings, parks & playgrounds